NO BULK!...for women
HOW TO GET (AND STAY THAT WAY) STRONGSLEEKFIT AND AGE 40 AND BEYOND!

iUniverse books may be ordered through booksellers or by contacting:

iUniverse
1663 Liberty Drive
Bloomington, IN 47403
www.iuniverse.com
1-800-Authors (1-800-288-4677)

ISBN: 978-1-6632-0004-4 (sc)
ISBN: 978-1-6632-0005-1 (e)

Library of Congress Control Number: 2020908470

Print information available on the last page.

iUniverse rev. date: 05/16/2020

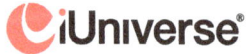

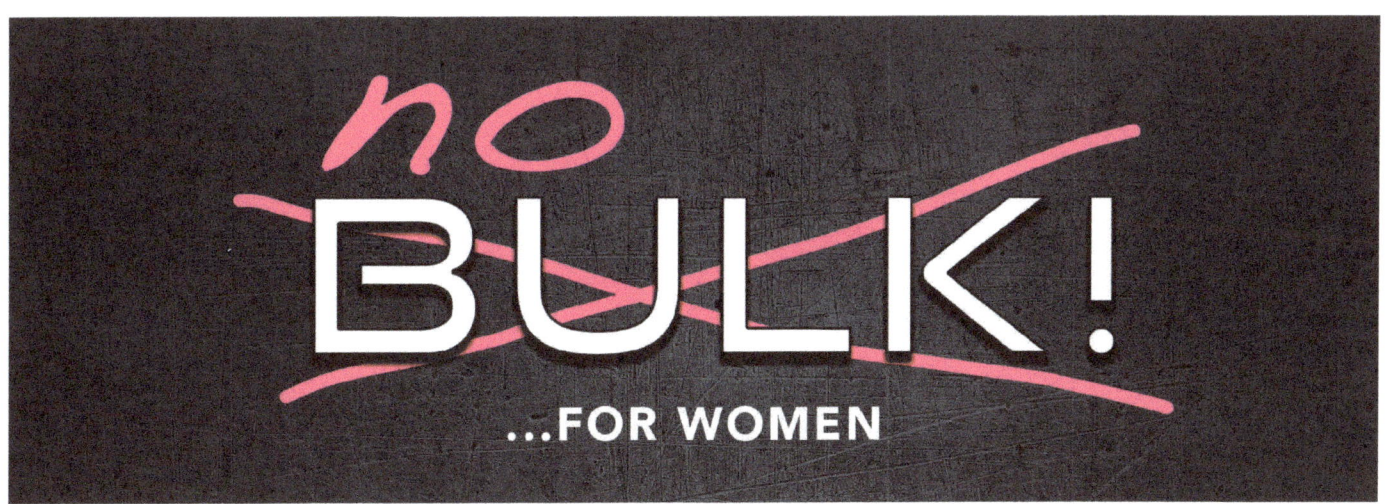

no
BULK!
...FOR WOMEN

by
Mister G

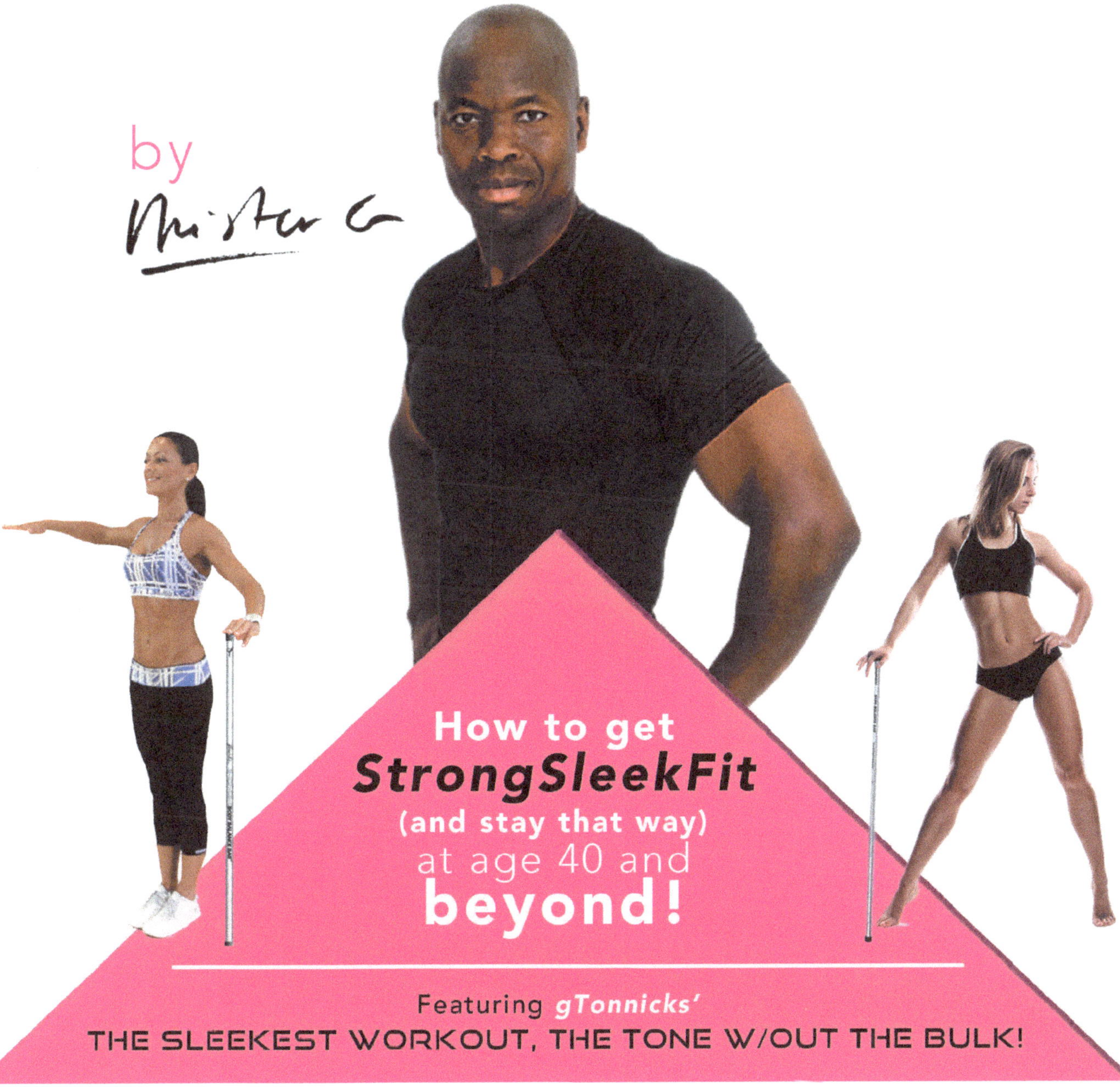

How to get
StrongSleekFit
(and stay that way)
at age 40 and
beyond!

Featuring *gTonnicks'*
THE SLEEKEST WORKOUT, THE TONE W/OUT THE BULK!

Mister G

- ARE YOU AFRAID OF BULKING UP WHEN LIFTING WEIGHTS OR JUST DON'T WANT TO GET TOO BIG?!!

- ARE YOU LOOKING FOR SOMETHING THAT WILL TARGET AND SHAPE UP YOUR ABS, HIPS, AND BUNS QUICKLY AND EFFECTIVELY?!

- WOULD YOU LIKE TO BUILD YOURSELF THAT STRONG & SLEEK PHYSIQUE THAT EVERYONE ADMIRES?

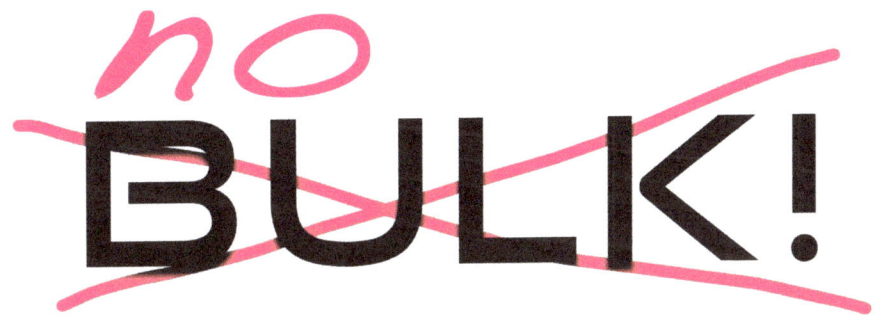

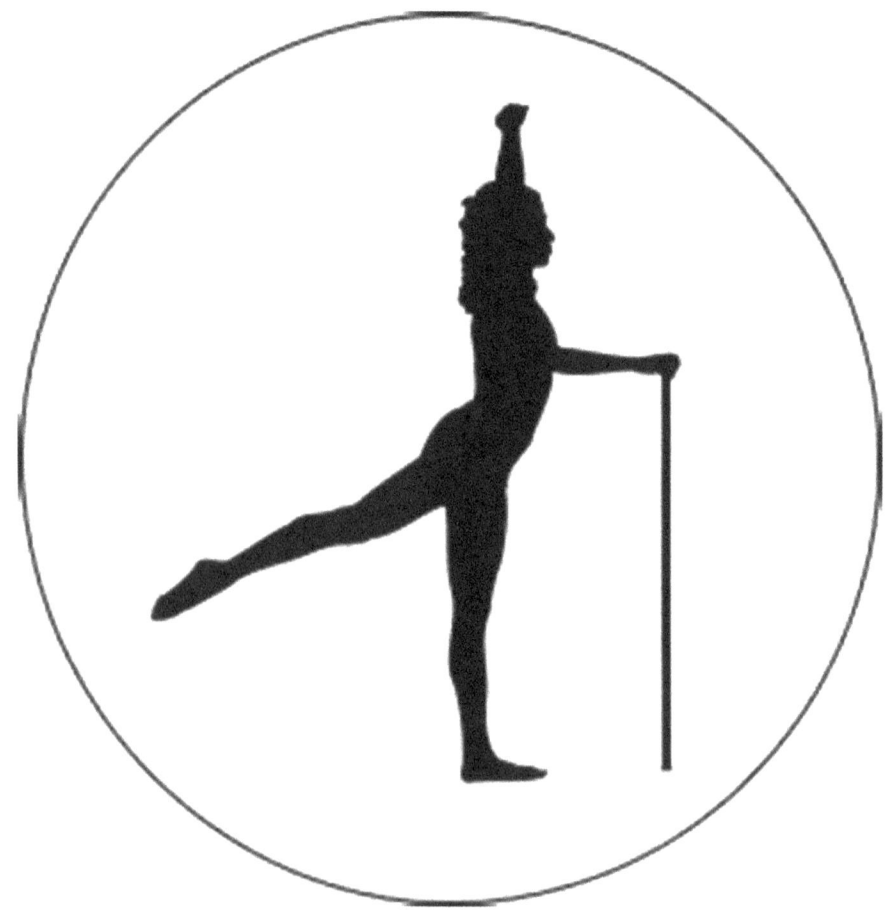

FOREWORD

"gTonnicks is more than just a workout, it's an expression of strength, elegance, and power."

Foreword from Garba "Mister G" Onadja

When I sat down to start writing this book it would be over nearly 35 years since I had been studying fitness and doing all kinds of workouts and physical conditioning as a former competitive athlete in various fields (Basketball, Soccer, Handball, Taekwondo, Wrestling, and Track & Field) while also, training and coaching various individuals, teams, and over 3 continents. My past and current clientele include executives, models, armed forces, celebrities, and other affluent personalities, and others from all walks of life.

While living in France in 1990 and observing Ballet dancers, La Savate (the French-style of kickboxing) practitioners and as a martial artist myself, I envisioned an exercise system that would be truly the essence of mind and body conditioning in its purest, most direct form. French Kickboxers move and execute their techniques with elegance, precision...and poise as if they were ballerinas, but in the ring. Ten years later, gTonnicks was born – a regimen incorporating the physical strength and mental discipline taught by these diverse mind & body conditioning forms I had observed earlier for years.

"gTonnicks is more than just a workout, it's an expression of strength, elegance, and power."

Utilizing my thirty plus years as a personal trainer, fitness instructor and martial artist, I had only one thing in mind when I created gTonnicks – to help my female clients, students and everyday people improve their overall tone and flexibility, while targeting the areas of the body that usually cause the most concern: the waist, abdomen, buns, and thighs.
I also wanted to help people achieve this without the risk of bulking up.

Foreword cont'd.

However, the best workout will fail to yield you the results you seek without proper nutrition. Since my adolescent years, I instinctively knew that food in conjunction with hormones and genetics, plays a crucial role in body shaping and athletic performance.

So ever since, I began studying more about sports nutrition trough books, fitness magazines and through my own observations and personal experiments. What I called the SleekFit Eating is the result of such accumulated experience throughout those years, which I'm now sharing with you.

I've made an intentional and deliberate effort to make this book as simple, straight forward, and to the point as much as possible without the usual lengthy, technical and scientifically complex explanation of most such written topics. The goal is for the reader to enjoy, understand the essentials and easily follow them. There are already countless available sources of comprehensive scientific information for those who want to verify or just learn more about any particular subject, statement, and other information in this book if they so choose. I've come to realize that people are more likely to read and apply information if they are readily made available to them in a simple and practical manner.

It will take you about 2 weeks to become familiar and implement the SleekFit Eating comfortably. During this learning and application phase, you will get to appreciate how simple and easy it is to follow. After those initial 2 weeks, you wouldn't even need to calculate anything anymore. You will only follow the portions as predetermined, except for occasional adjustments as your body shapes up nicely. This is precisely what this book is all about as it also introduces gTonnicks and features gTonnicks' The Sleekest Workout program.

PART 1: INTRODUCING gTONNICKS' "THE SLEEKEST WORKOUT" PROGRAM

"A goal without a plan is just a wish"

Part 1: Introducing gTonnicks' *"The Sleekest Workout" Program*

- **Are you afraid of bulking up when lifting weights or just don't want to get too big?!!**

- **Are you looking for something that will target and shape up your abs, hips, and buns quickly and effectively?!**

- **Would you like to build yourself that strong & sleek physique that everyone admires?**

Find out all about what Hollywood celebrities, models, dancers, and others are doing to stay fit and sleek: gTonnicks' *"The Sleekest Workout"™*! It's the most powerful and most effective strength & toning video ever created to make you *StrongSleekFit™* It has all those benefits at once: total body strength & tone, endurance, cardio, stretch, including abs, hips & buns shaping!

gTonnicks' *"The Sleekest Workout"™* is based on the most innovative, most powerful, strength training program on the market today, *gTonnicks®!*

When it comes to Abs, Hips & Buns, NOTHING hit those muscles as effectively and efficiently as *gTonnicks®!*

gTonnicks® was created by L.A.'s premier trainer and 10th degree Master Black Belt, Garba "Mister G" Onadja. Voted "most motivating fitness instructor" by the DAILY NEWSPAPER readers and praised as Calabasas Top Personal Trainer & Fitness Motivator.

gTonnicks' The Sleekest Workout consists of two (phases 1 & 2) full body workout routines and two targeted workout routines for the abs and the hips & gluteus.

One Workout Gives You All These Benefits ...at Once!

- Toning & Strengthening
- Fat Burning
- Core Building
- Hips & Buns Shaping
- And More!

What Is gTonnicks?

gTonnicks is an innovative (machine-free) approach to body strengthening, toning, and stretching using mainly the gBalance Bar. gTonnicks can also be described as high-precision toning because it can isolate practically any muscle for optimum toning and strength, including the core muscles and especially the so-called "hard-to-reach" areas such as abs, hips, buns and (inner) thighs. Additionally, gTonnicks stresses "No wasted movements"; utilizing the most compelling force in the universe – gravity – in conjunction with body weight, to aid in resistance training.

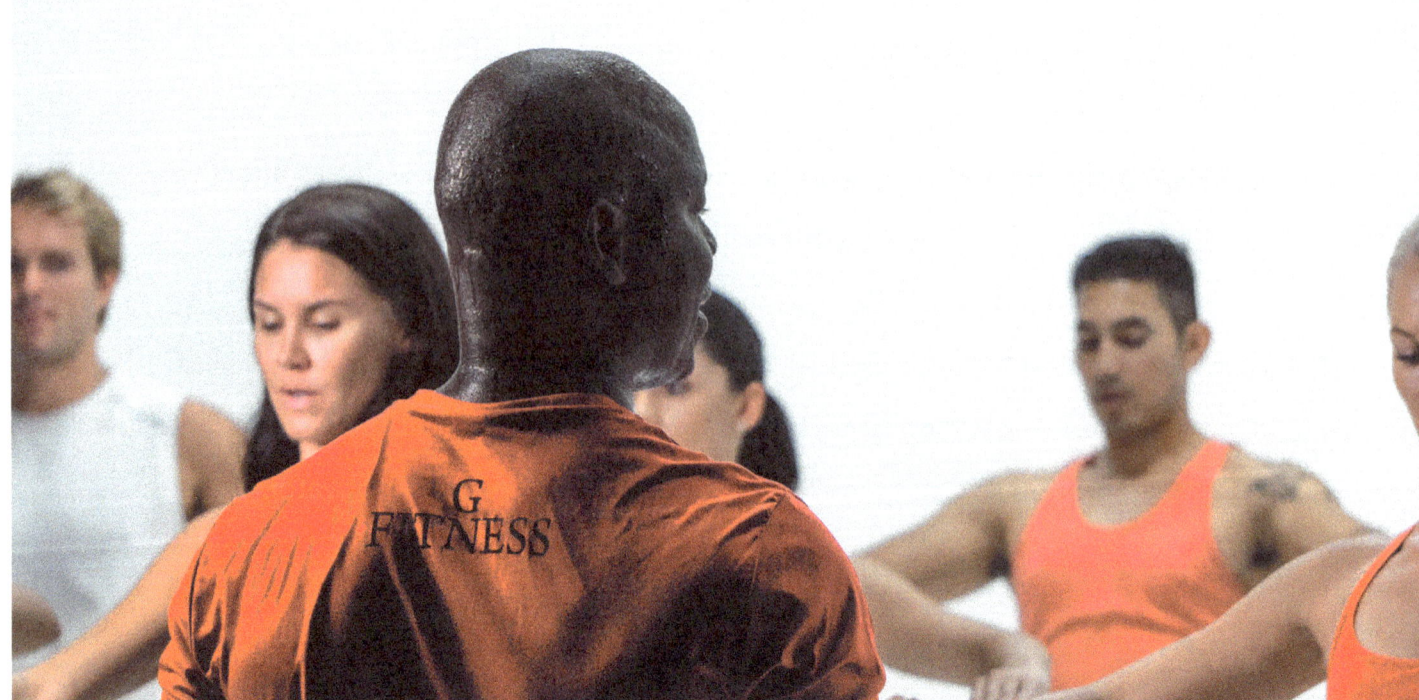

Below is one of the gTonnicks signature moves called Arabesque Leg Lift.

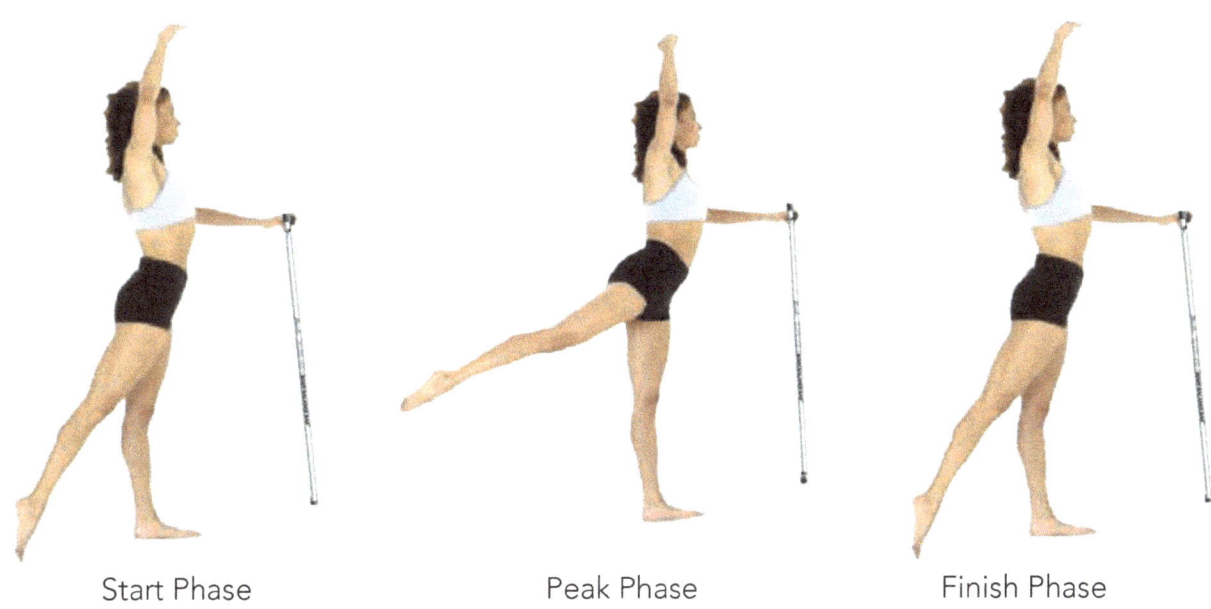

Start Phase   Peak Phase   Finish Phase

Also, gTonnicks movements are performed in a relatively slow motion with regard to form, balance, precision, breathing and body alignment (correct posture), thus, forcing the participant to concentrate and focus on the movement. That's one of the reasons we consider gTonnicks as the only Power-Toning™ System in the world!

The beauty of gTonnicks emanates from the fact that the exercises are executed in the same scientifically precise sequences that dancers, gymnasts, some martial artists, and other superbly toned athletes use to build and maintain the physiques we all envy and admire.

A Workout Like No Other

I can fairly state with almost certainty that you've never experienced with any other workout what you're about to experience with gTonnicks. That's because gTonnicks is essentially based on the Intentional and Purposeful Contraction of the Muscle, or IPCM along with the utilization of the gBalance Bar, and other fundamental principles.

Below is the Front Leg Extension exercise in gTonnicks, which primarily works the quadriceps (front thigh muscles).

gTonnicks Leg Front Extension:

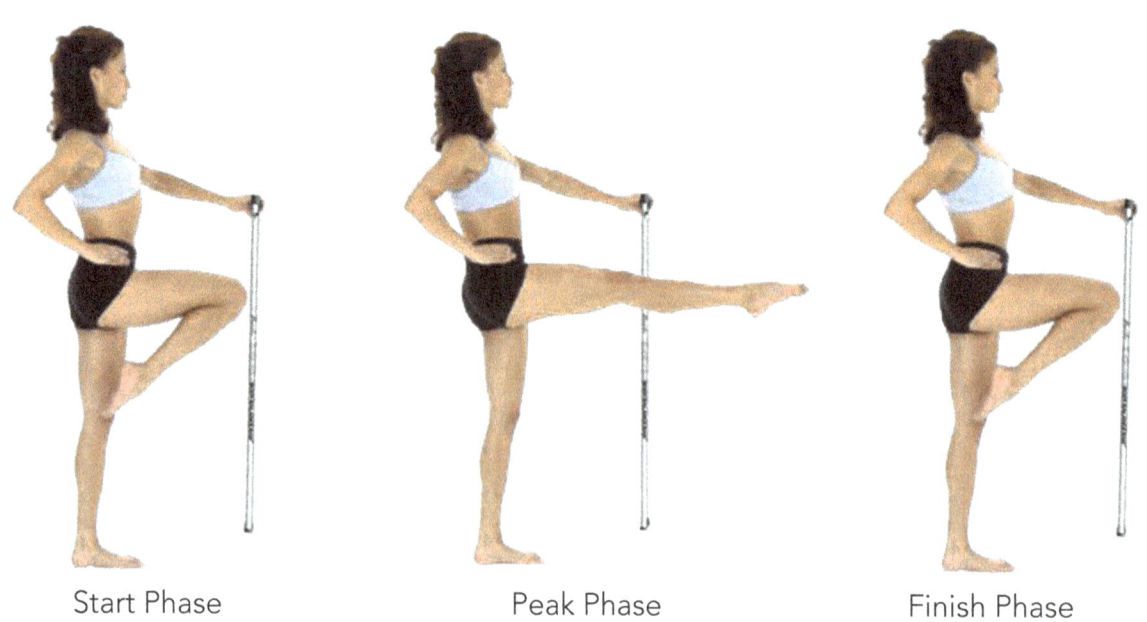

Start Phase   Peak Phase   Finish Phase

Intentional and Purposeful Contraction of the Muscle (IPCM)

The IPCM requires you to contract your muscles (especially the abs) right at the beginning of each move and maintain that contraction throughout. As a result, gTonnicks makes you sweat with benefits such as increase in body temperature or heart rate upon which are indicators of increased metabolic rate, accelerated energy expenditure, and increased lipid oxidation (fat burning) from neuromuscular activation.

The gBalance Bar

Every move in gTonnicks emanates from the core and starts with the contraction of the muscles. The gBalance Bar (gBB) is an integral part of gTonnicks that obliges you to activate your core muscles as it serves for "balance check" rather than something to hold on to like you would do with crutch. As simple as it is, the gBalance Bar (gBB) might be the most powerful fitness tool.

A POWERFUL TOOL THAT FORCES THE ACTIVATION OF THE CORE MUSCLES.

The use of the gBalance Bar helps:

- *Incite the core muscles.*
- *Improve posture.*
- *Promote proper form.*
- *Increase body control.*
- *Improve focus & concentration.*
- *You get in tune with your body better.*
- *Make your workout overall much better.*
- *With much more!*

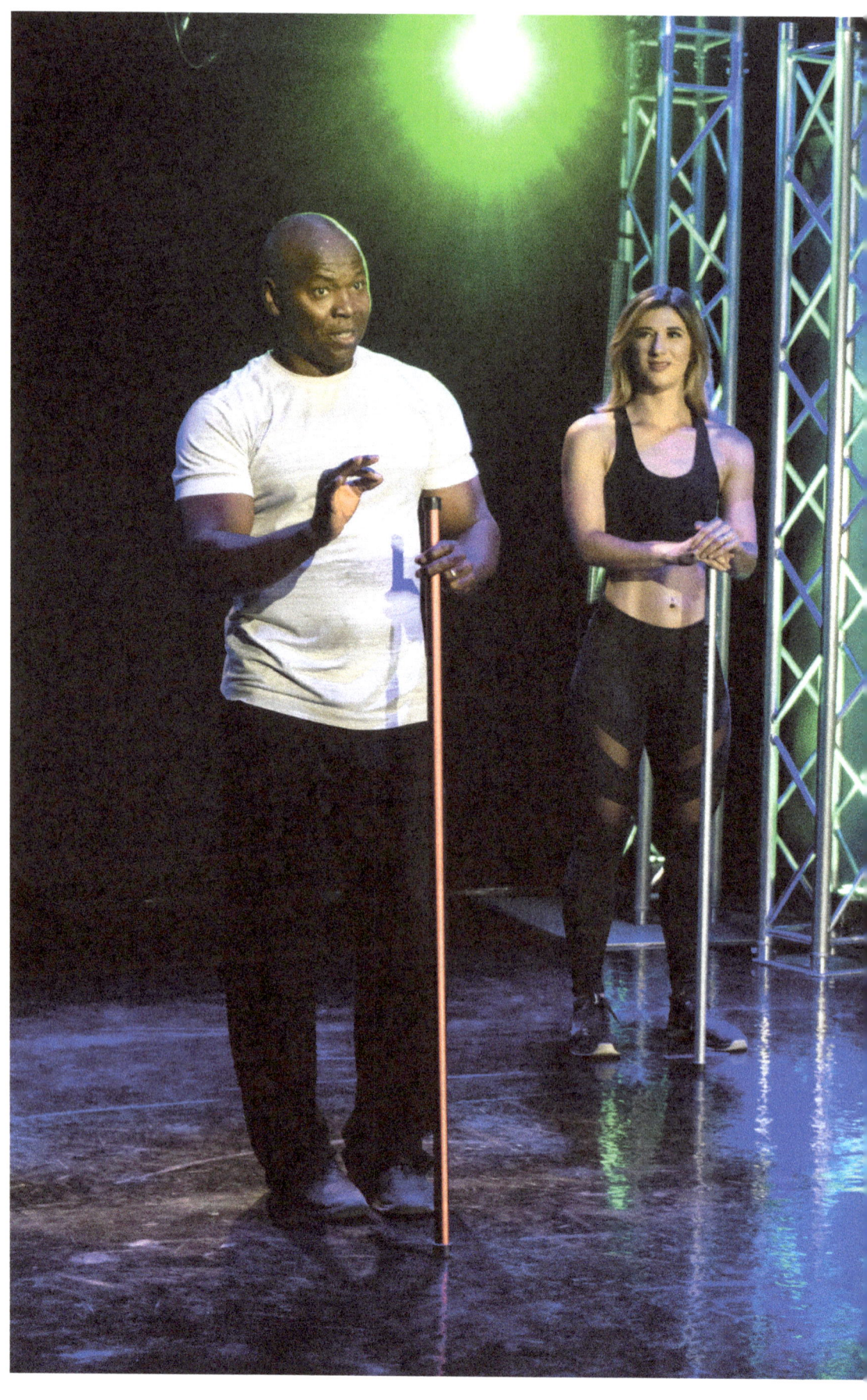

AS SIMPLE AS IT IS,

THE gBALANCE BAR (gBB)

MIGHT BE THE MOST POWERFUL FITNESS TOOL.

The gBalance Bar is made of aluminum with a smooth coating and a sleek design. It comes in two parts to be screwed tight together to form a single unit bar. There is a 42 inch-long gBalance Bar and a 48 inch-long one. The 42 inch-long gBalance Bar are meant for individuals who are about 5'6" tall or less and the 48 inch-long gBalance Bar for those who are about 5'7" tall or more.

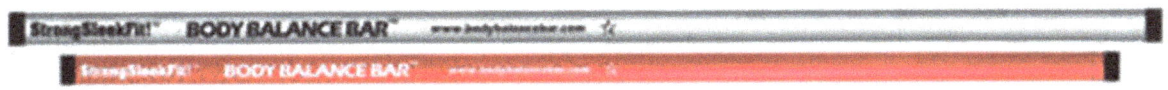

The Tone Without the Bulk

If Bodybuilders grow bigger muscles by applying the progressive load (lifting heavier and heavier weights) technique as they do, including eating more, it's fairly accurate to assess that bulk can be avoided with limited progressive load and food intake, and by using bodyweight and gravity as natural resistance for optimum strength & tone. Simply watch the many athletes such as martial artists, gymnasts, track & fielders, ballerinas and other sport performers with the superb bodies they've developed as a result of their training. Most of them spend a minimum time in the weight room as the majority of their body conditioning is based on bodyweight and other natural resistance such as gravity and other elements of nature. Don't give me wrong, I'm not against lifting weights. On the contrary, I'm a big advocate of weightlifting and spend a great deal of time in the gym myself, but only after my competitive years in Taekwondo, soccer, basketball, and other sports.

During those years, I was as strong, sleek, and as fit as I could be. My physical conditioning was mostly composed of bodyweight exercises such as push-ups, pull-ups, stretching, and other functional athletic exercises like sprints, hoping, and plyometrics. I only started to lift more weights after I was done with competition and wanting to bulk up a bit. Weightlifting, especially with free weights (e.g. barbells, dumbbells) are great ways to build strength, fix strength imbalances, and increase muscle size in desired areas of the body. It just has to be done appropriately. Nonetheless, I can tell you right now that weightlifting has little to nothing to do with athletic power. Ask Simon Biles (the gymnastic phenomenon), Hussein Bolt (the Jamaican sprinters), Michael Jordan, or the Volleyball champion Gabrielle Reece. None of them credit weightlifting for their sports prowess. Neither do I for my own athletic achievements. I'm a former multiple champion in Taekwondo and basketball. If weightlifting was a big factor in athletic performance, bodybuilders would be shattering all records in sports. Instead, most of them couldn't even run to save their lives. That's a story for another time. For the time being, just know that core strength development, which differs from bodybuilding is actually the foundation for athletic power. Core strength is what gTonnicks evolves from.

gTonnicks and your Body

The entire gTonnicks system evolves from three of its fundamental and most powerful principles.

Principle # 1: Intentional and purposeful contraction (IPCM) of the muscle.

Principle # 2: Core strength applied. It's one thing to have core strength and another to apply it. gTonnicks accomplishes both simultaneously.

Principle # 3: Natural free body motion with combined gravity and bodyweight for resistance.

The application of these gTonnicks principles allows for:

- *Tone without bulking up*
- *Core strength development*
- *Reach of any muscle directly and effectively*
- *Body control & balance*
- *Functionality*

Now, you may ask: why focusing on the muscle?

There are many reasons. Here are some of them:

- *The muscle burns fat the most*
- *The muscle consumes the most calories*
- *The muscle moves the body.*
- *The muscle increases metabolism*
- *The muscle protects the bones and other organs.*
- *The muscle allows blood circulation and oxygenation.*
- *The muscle enhances athletic performance.*
- *The muscle softens the skin.*
- *The muscle keeps the body young.*
- *The muscle increases sensuality.*

Now, I ask you: how many people have you seen (you might even be one of them) lose weight by doing only cardio or simply dieting only to realize how weak and flabby her/his body is? How loose her or his skin is? That's caused by lack of muscle work. A big reason why I introduced gTonnicks to my clients and members of my gym back in 1998 is precisely because they complained about not feeling toned in spite of their weight loss.

During that time, cardio was the main mode of workout for most. The truth is, focusing on the muscle like gTonnicks does, makes everything you do more effective and more enjoyable. You burn more calories on your cardio and burn fat throughout your day and even at sleep.

It's a scientifically proven fact!

What Makes gTonnicks So Exceptionally Effective

• Intentional and purposeful muscle contraction – gTonnicks utilizes your body for resistance and toning in addition to voluntarily muscle contraction before and throughout every move, thus maximizing strength & toning, including calorie burning.

• No muscle is out of reach – Behind every move there is a specific muscle or set of muscles involved. By using free natural and functional motions, gTonnicks allows you to work and tone any muscle you desire – including those hard-to-reach manage and develop ones like hips, buttocks, thighs and abdomen.

• The dynamic pause – gTonnicks "dynamic pause" maximizes muscular intensity via isometric contraction of all the whole body for a brief period of time.

Controlled and precise movements – gTonnicks requires precision and control, which increases efficiency and effectiveness in working the targeted muscles.

• The body as the machine – gTonnicks primary uses bodyweight and gravity as natural resistance thus, making the body simultaneously the means and the goal.

More on gTonnicks

• Hate it. Love it! I would be the first one to admit my "love / hate" relationship with gTonnicks. I "hate" it because I know it will kick my you-know-what and in a hurry (I mean within moments) and I love it because of well… the exact same reason I hate it. So, I just would like you to think of the experience gTonnicks like your first taste of something tonic like coffee, tea, or an exotic fruit that's good for you. You will feel its strong tone right away as it "hits" you, but then develop a taste and appreciation for it overtime.

• Don't be fooled. gTonnicks workout is quite something else. Simple, yet so effective. Looks easy, yet so intense. You will feel the toning effects immediately and the muscle fatigue rather quickly. It's all good, though. It's gTonnicks!

But, just don't take my word for it. Try those gTonnicks moves following the instructions and see for yourself:

Quiz:

QUESTION:

Why do most seemingly fit-looking men hate gTonnicks?

ANSWER:

Because it humbles them.

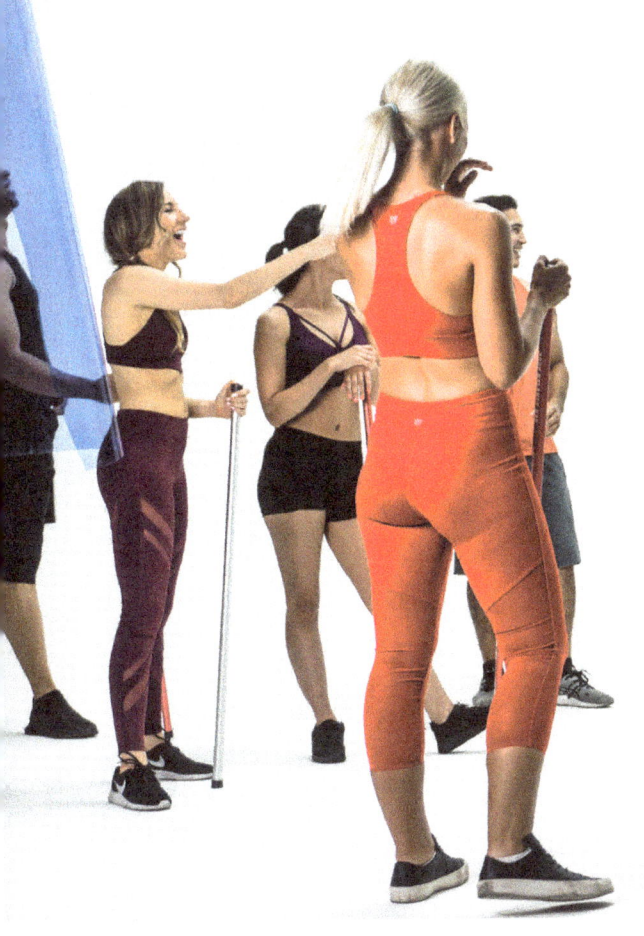
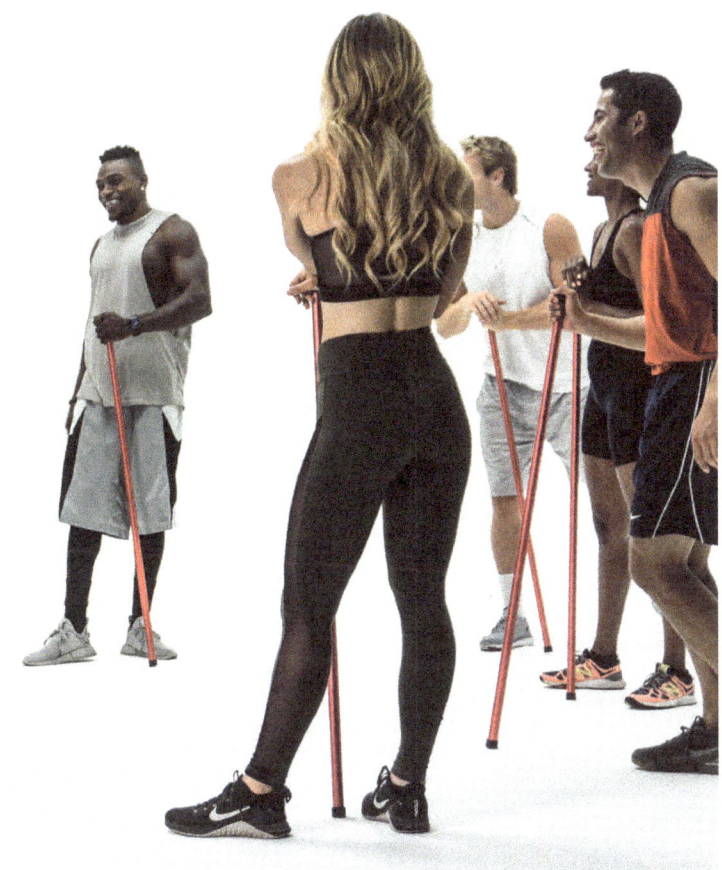

Front Straight Leg Raises

Target Areas: Primarily targets the quads and hip flexors.

Secondary targets: abdomen/calves.

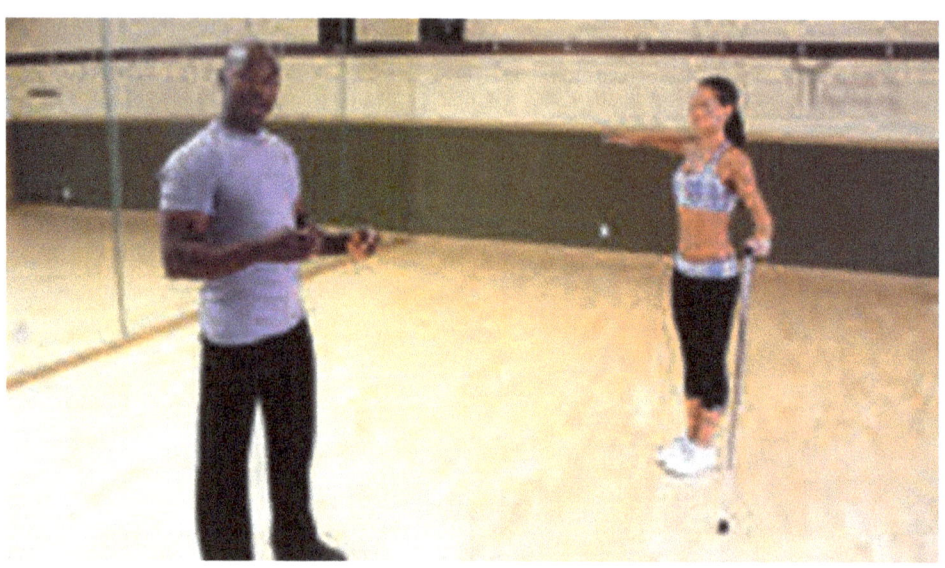

PROCEDURE:

Raise foot off the floor to waist level, or as high as possible. Hold abdominal in and slightly tight. You raise and lower the leg, keeping it stiff, so the muscles never relax. Pointing toes in will work the shin muscles. Exhale while going down – inhale while going up.

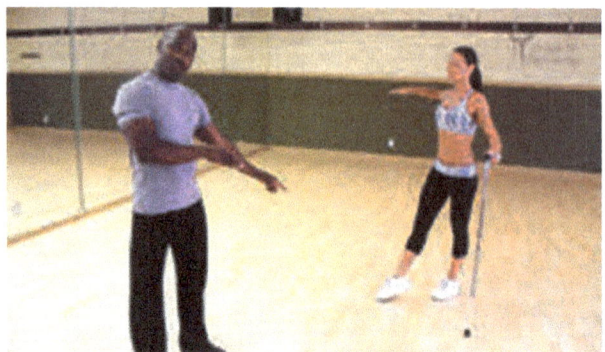
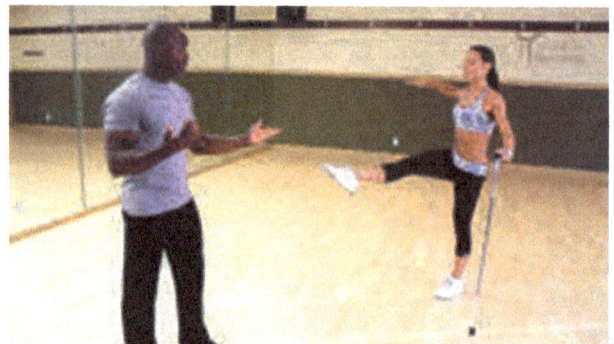

Ballet Squat

Target Areas: Primarily targets the thigh muscles.

Secondary targets are the upper/lower back.

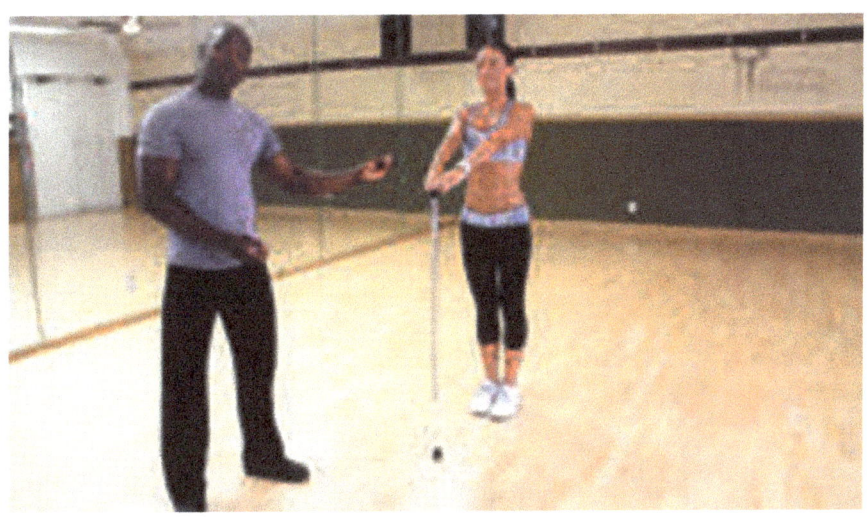

PROCEDURE:

Start with feet wide apart in a "martial arts" stance and slightly turned out. Hold the BBB in front of you at arm's length in a vertical position by the fingertips. Your feet should be slightly wider than shoulder width apart, but in the same direction, not angled. Move hips slowly down, but not more than 90 degrees from the floor. Make sure knees are wide. Exhale while going down – inhale while going up.

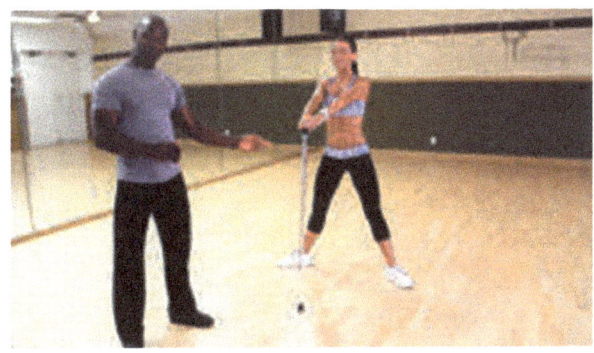
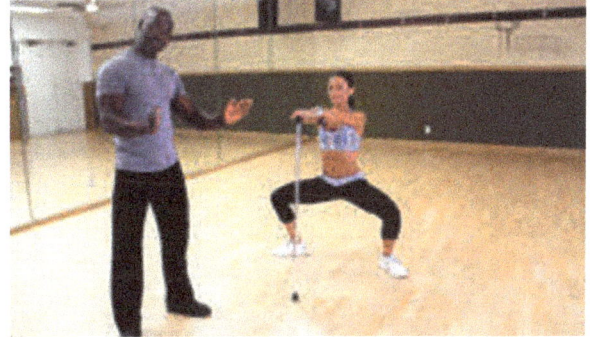

Side Leg Raises

Target Areas: Primarily targets the hips, obliques and gluteus.

Secondary targets: adductors.

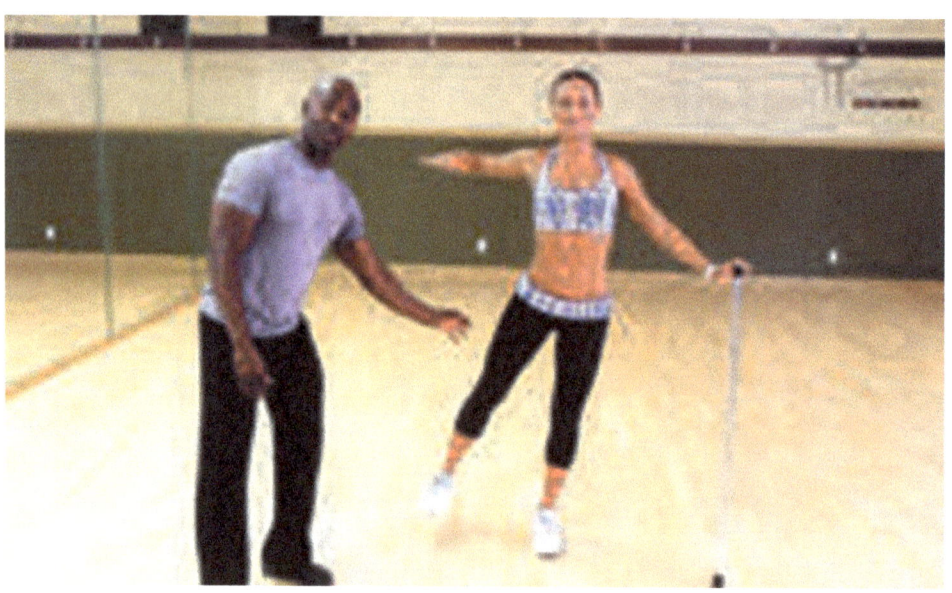

PROCEDURE:

You start with your foot off the floor and yourbody straight up. Toes should be pointed up, flexing the angle. Lift the leg using the strength of the oblique muscles and hips. As you reach the highest level, you want to turn the toes slightly downward, making the gluteus and hips work more. Exhale while going down – inhale while going up.

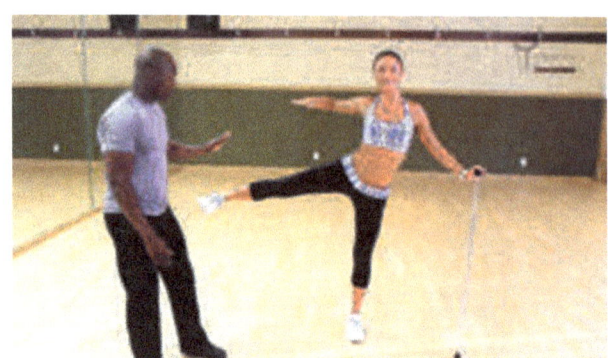
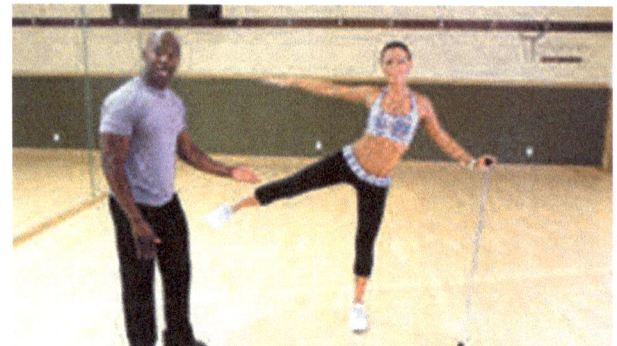

How to use gTonnicks' The Sleekest Workout program

gTonnicks' The Sleekest Workout consists of two (phases 1 & 2) full body workout routines and two targeted workout routines for the abs and the hips & gluteus.

Then, there is the SleekFit eating plan

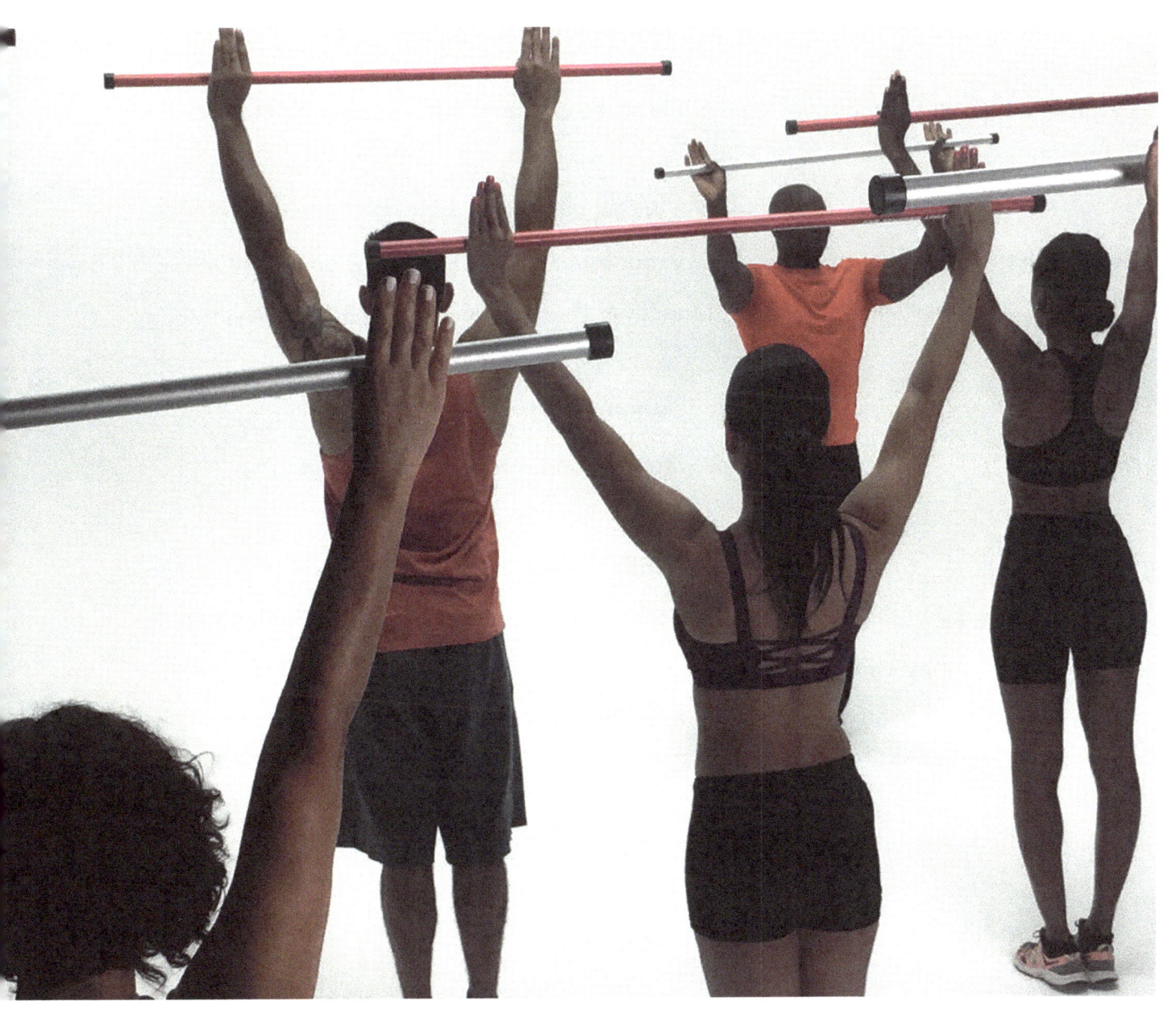

The routine in the gTonnicks' The Sleekest Workout package includes 4 different workout routines:

1. **Full Body Tone Phase 1 (30 - 50 minutes long)**
2. **Full Body Tone Phase 2 (30 - 50 minutes long)**
3. **PureAbs routine (12 - 20 minutes - bonus)**
4. **PureHips & Buns routine (12 - 20 minutes - bonus)**

This is a 12-week long training schedule at the end of which, you shall be StrongSleekFit!

WEEK ONE

Begin with the Full Body Tone Phase 1 workout routine. Do it twice only on Week One with 2 days

break in between (e.g. Monday & Thursday or Tuesday & Saturday)

WEEK TWO

Repeat Week One with the same workout and off days.

WEEK THREE

Add a day of the Full Body Tone workout routine and take your workout schedule

from twice weekly to 3 times a week on either M/W/F or T/Th/S,

which gives you a rest day on the alternate days.

WEEK FOUR

Repeat Week Three with the exact same workout schedule.

WEEK FIVE

Continue with the 3x weekly Full Body Tone Phase 1 workout routine. However, add a minimum-impact cardio activity (e.g. walking, cycling, or gliding on an elliptical machine) on two of the alternate days (Tuesday & Thursday or Monday & Friday) and or 20 to 60 minutes. Tip: the lesser the duration, the brisker the activity should be. You may do those cardio activities either indoor or outdoor.

WEEK SIX

Add another cardio activity day onto your Week Five workout schedule M/F/W or T/Th/S. Use Sundays for rest and to rejuvenate your body with a stretching routine like the one provided in the gTonnicks Unlimited Series Streaming. Aim to achieve 15 repetitions on all 3 rounds in all 3 days of the week.

WEEK SEVEN

Start the Full Body Tone Phase 2 workout routine with the same workout schedule as the one in Week Three, including the cardio activities and so on. Aim to achieve 15 repetitions on all 3 rounds in all 3 days of the week by Week 12.

NOTE: *The Full Body Tone workout routine can be found in the OnDemand page of The Sleekest Workout. Use your Access Code from your purchase of the gBalance Bar.*

OPTIONAL: *The PureAbs and the PureHips&Buns workout routines are optional. If you feel like hitting those areas abs or gluteus some more, do them on your cardio days right before the cardio!*

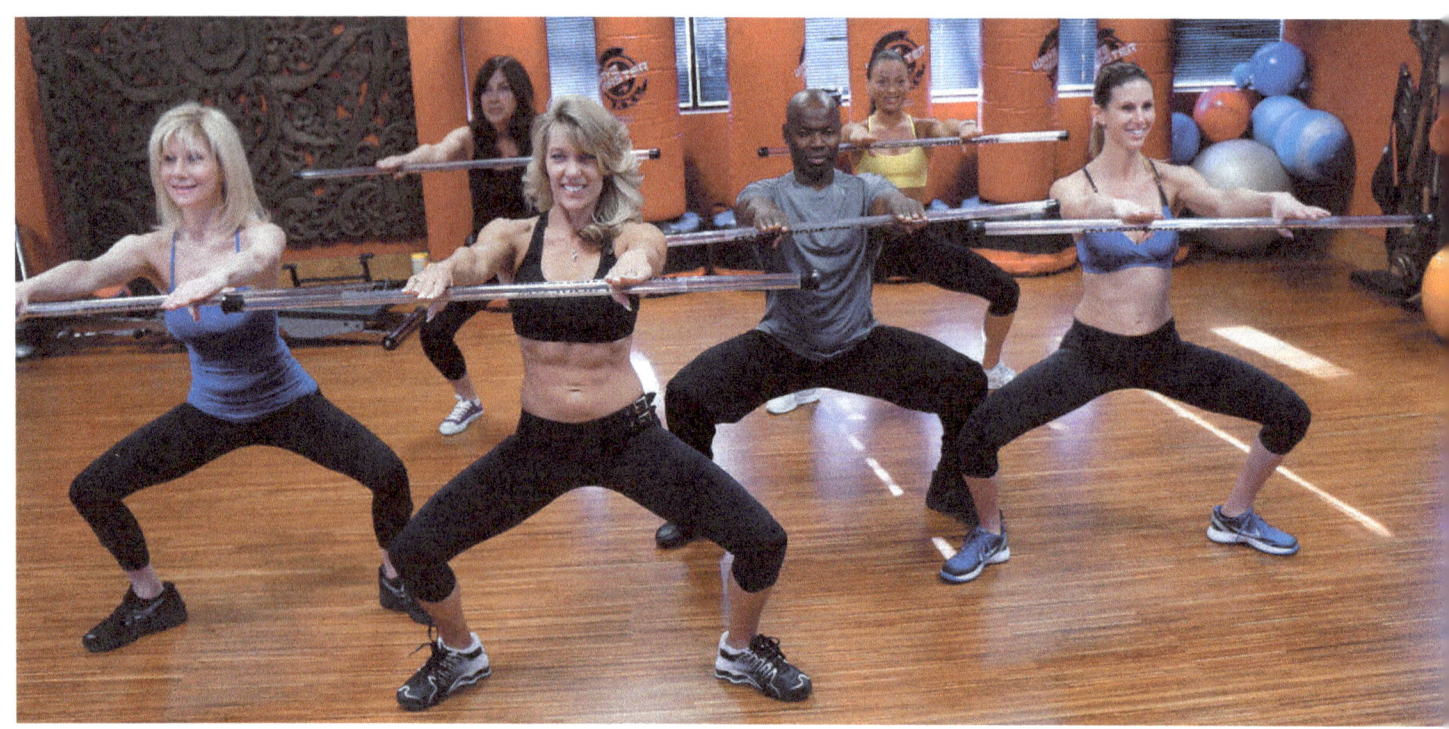

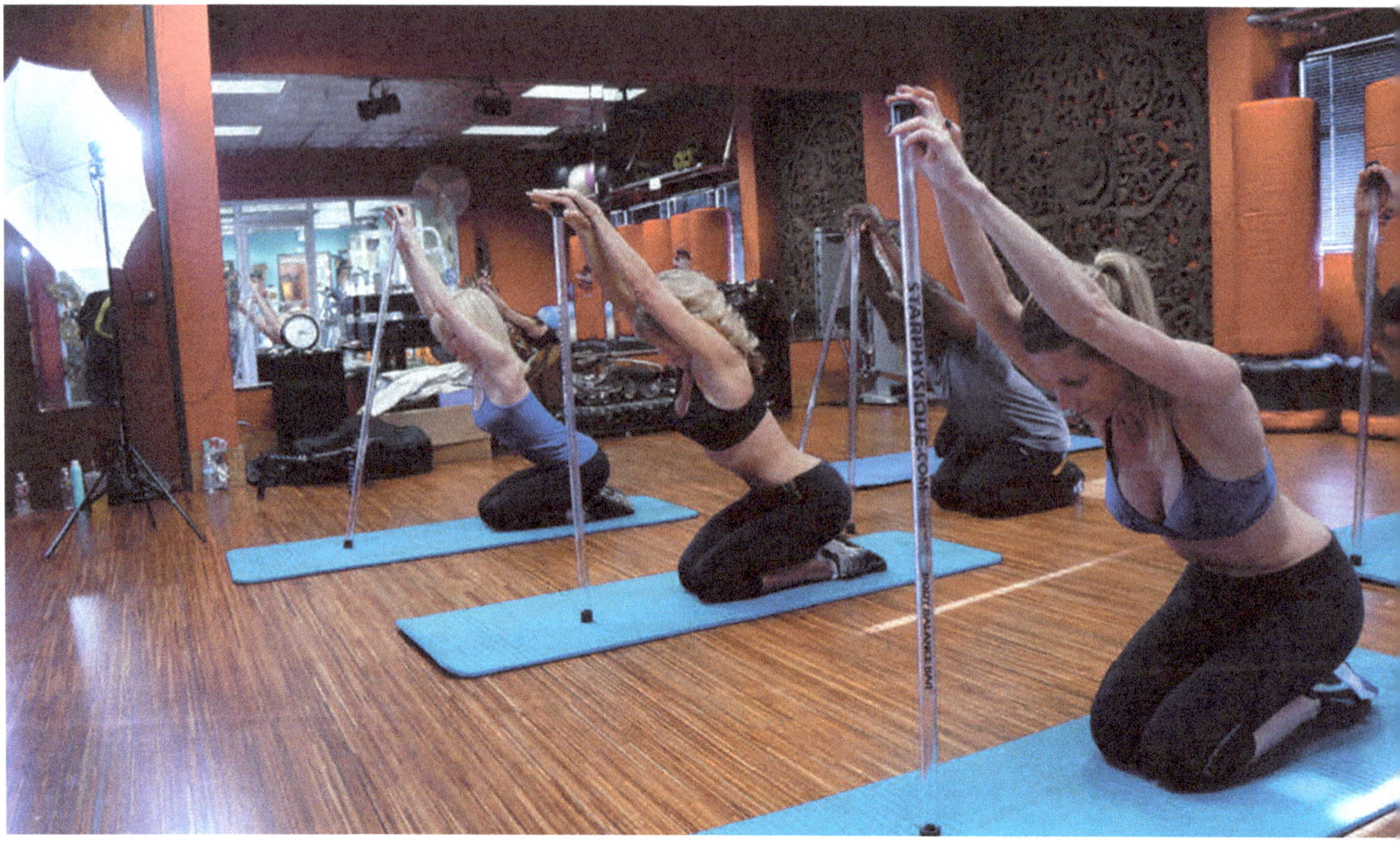

NOTIFICATION: *as the owner of this book, you're entitled to access the workout streaming video. You will need to purchase the gBalance Bar in order to do the workout effectively. Please go to TheSleekestWorkout.com or gTonnickStyle.com to purchase the gBalance Bar. Upon purchase, you will receive and access code to the video streaming via your email address.*

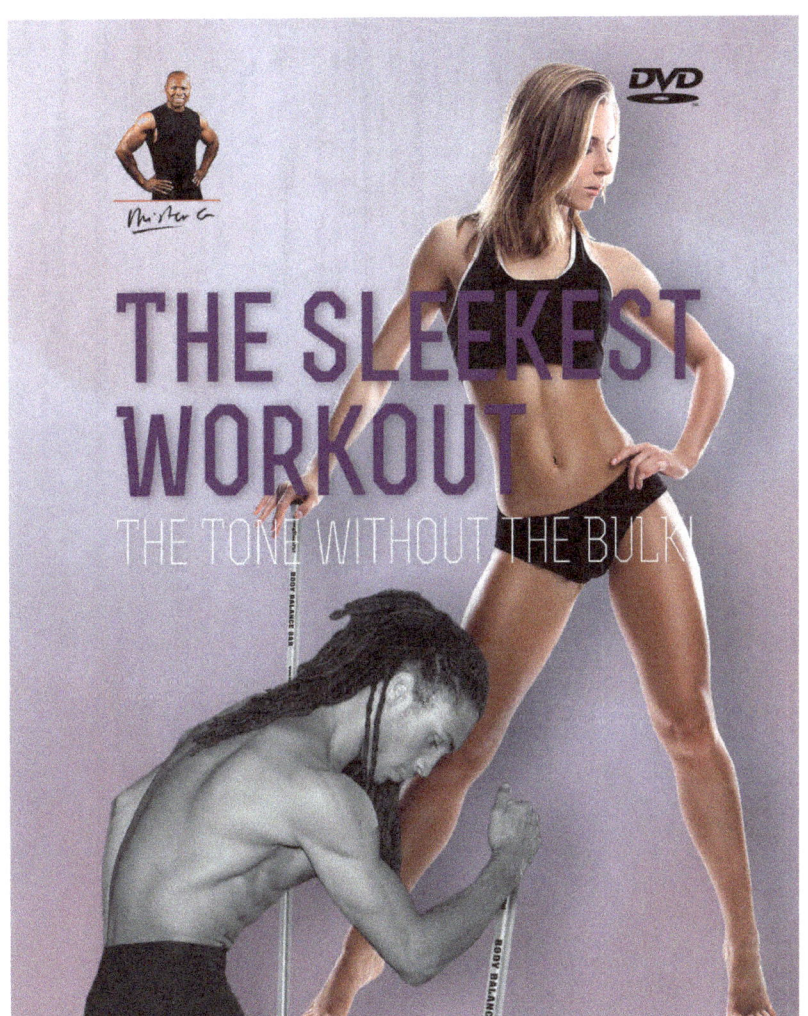

The best way to lose weight is by combining appropriate eating with proper exercising and no workout uses the body to work the body as gTonnicks. No exercise regimen shapes up the body and the mind as genetically, organically, naturally, and powerfully as gTonnicks.

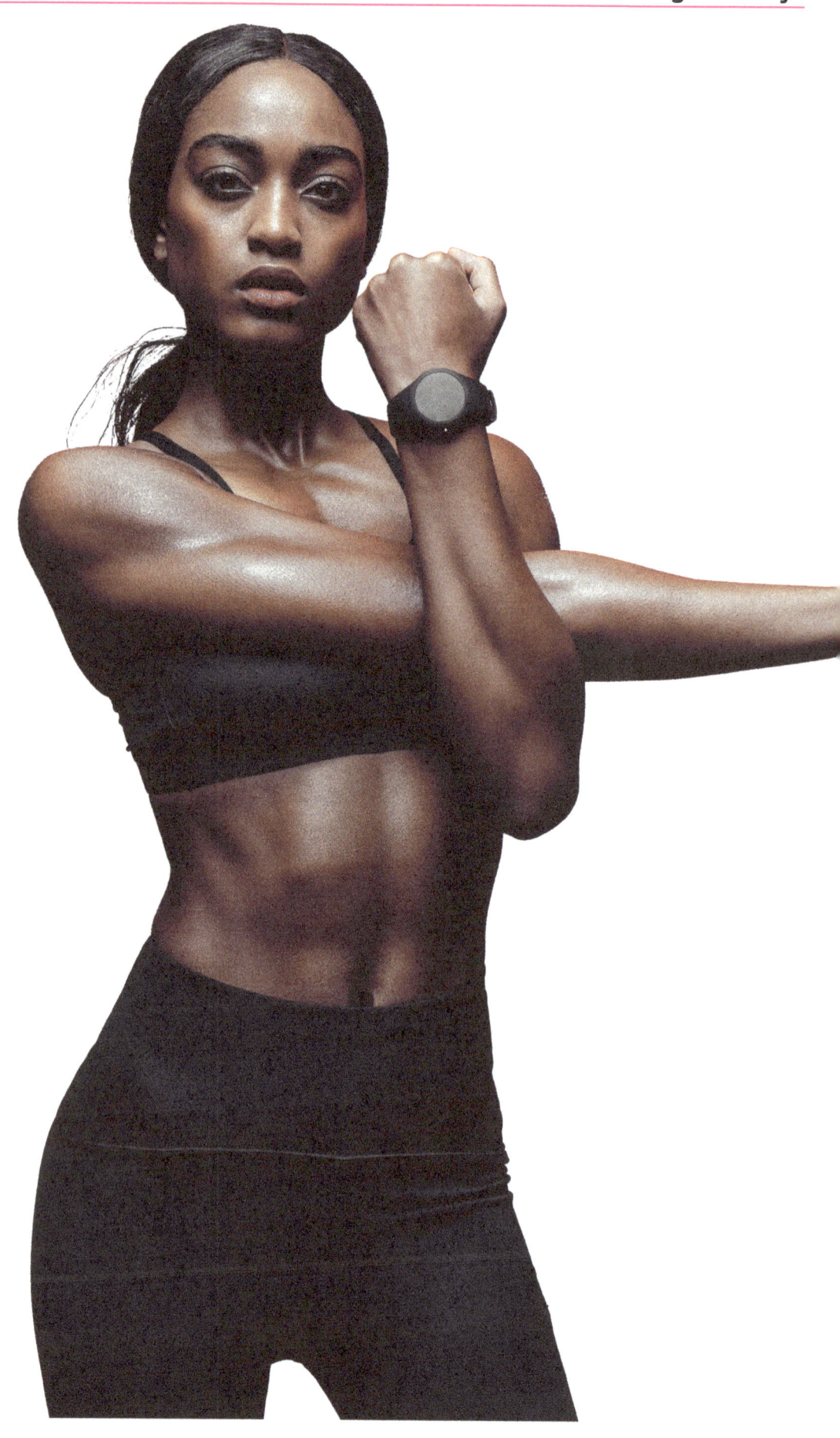

PART 2: UNDERSTANDING THE BODY

"Take care of your body, it's the only place you have to live in"

Part 2: Understanding the Body

Now that we know a little more about gTonnicks and its effects on the body, let's talk about the body itself, the types of bodies, including strength and metabolism.

Body Genetics & Metabolism

There are three general categories of body types: ectomorph, mesomorph, and endomorph. Each body type determines the metabolism for that body type. Metabolism is the rate at which the body processes food and burn calories.

• The ectomorph is described lean and long with difficulty building muscle, which means it has a very high metabolism. An individual with such genetic type tends not to gain weight in spite of eating anything and as much as desired. Skip a meal and you might disappear if you're an ectomorph.

• The endomorph is built more on the thick side with greater tendency to store fat. He or she can be pear-shaped, or thick overall. The endomorph type seems like he or she can put weight on by simply smelling food.

• The mesomorph is the athletic and well-built type with a high metabolism and responsive muscle cells. Rub yourself against a dumbbell if you're a mesomorph, and you grow muscle instantly.

It's important that you understand which body type might be yours and how it fits in the equation of getting it sleek. That is lean and toned. However, beware that only very few people fall perfectly into one of the three categories. In fact, it has become increasingly difficult to distinguish the endomorph from the mesomorph thanks to the crappy American food. Seriously. As I write this paragraph News just break that half of the American population will be obese in 10 years. That's in year 2030! Not far away. Increasing number of children are getting obese too. It is my general understanding that whatever body type you have and keep for at least 2 years after you hit puberty is your body type. It's hard to tell nowadays as bad nutrition skews it all. Too many children are already overweight by the time they reach puberty. It's hard to tell the body type with this plague. Lifestyle and environment do affect genetics after all. You are what you eat. So, most people are somewhere in between body types.

Fortunately, nature is not a precise science. It is in constant change and evolution, which actually is a good thing because it means that people can improve their physical appearance and sway themselves more towards the desired body type. That's right. Even genetics can be influenced by the environment and lifestyle thanks to the power of adaption (nature nurtures) for survival. gTonnicks' the Sleekest Workout program attempts to do just that with your genetics.

Determining body genetics

The ectomorph body type has shoulders that are narrower than the hips with fitted jeans generally feeling loose around your butt. The forearms are on the smallish side. The body tends to stay skinny by default and often long and narrow. If the ectomorph grips his or her wrist between the thumb and middle finger, the 2 fingers overlap.
Endomorphs generally have a smooth, round body, medium-large bone structure, small shoulders and shorter limbs. They usually carry their weight in the lower abdomen, hips, and thighs rather than evenly distributed throughout the body.

People with a mesomorph body type tend to have a medium frame. They may develop muscles easily and have more muscle than fat on their bodies. Mesomorphs are typically strong and solid. Not overweight or underweight. Their bodies may be described as rectangular in shape with an upright posture.

CAUTION: nature is not a "precise" science. It's rather a complex science in constant evolution and changes; that's the beauty of it. So, do not let yourself get bogged down into "fitting" in exactly into any of those body types, for as mentioned earlier very few people fit perfectly in any of those body types!

Metabolism

So, metabolism is the process by which the body converts food into useable energy in order to function and to keep itself alive. In general, the denser your muscles, the higher your metabolism because muscles are the biggest consumers of calories. So, the more you use your muscles, the more calories you burn. The toner you get, the more effectively you burn fat even at rest, especially following a strength and tone workout like gTonnicks.

The Basic Metabolic Rate (BMR) and Energy Expenditure Requirements (EER).

If metabolism is the rate at which the body processes food for energy, the basic metabolic rate (BMR) is the minimum amount of that energy (or calories) the body needs to sustain itself with minimum activity. The BMR can also be interpreted as the estimated energy requirement (EER) with the understanding that the EER usually relates to a specific activity beyond the minimum such as exercising and other physically demanding activity. How to determine your BMR and EER will be explained later in this book.

Core Strength and Functionality

There are somewhat 625 muscles in the body. The main function of the muscle is to create movement, which means that for every move or moves there is a specific muscle or set of muscles involved as either prime movers, stabilizers, or neutralizers. The muscle also serves as protective layer for the skeleton and other internal organs.

Core strength is actually the very basis of physical strength and athleticism; they involve the very muscles from which power flows to the rest of the body. These muscles cover the core areas of the body, the trunk, the spine, and the abdominal wall, to which they are all attached. The core muscles primarily work as stabilizers and neutralizers for the body and assist the primary muscle movers such as the biceps during exercises like the standing arm curls, or the quadriceps in a squat exercise. Any good martial artist, or athlete can easily assess the necessity of such areas in the power center for athletic performance. In my twenty years as a personal trainer and fitness instructor, I am yet to meet someone who truly understands core strength and how to use it fully. In the last five years, I have not spent a training session without reminding my clients to tighten the abdominal area at least 20 times! They simply keep forgetting to use those muscles; however, they always recognize the difference it makes when they do use them as they do every time with gTonnicks. gTonnicks, which teaches how to utilize those very core muscles most advantageously in lifting more weights safely. We will get to gTonnicks' The Sleekest Workout program later in this book.

Functionality of the body is simply its suitability to perform practical daily activities such as bending, climbing, lifting or carrying objects around, including the in-house or yard work. Such body functionality also involves sport activities. gTonnicks uses natural biomechanics and functional moves to strength and tone every muscle of the body, thus this free and unrestricted set of motions not only leaves no muscle out of reach, but it also works the muscle to its optimum development.

Strength Training and Muscle Hypertrophy

Muscular hypertrophy is often associated with a strength-development program. This hypertrophy is the result of an increase in the size of individual muscle cells. Bodybuilders surely know how to build themselves bigger muscles and bulkier bodies. One of the training principles – they're many of them – and most popular one is what's called progressive loading, which consists of adding more load (weights) to lift overtime as the subject adapts and gets stronger through consistence training. Another element is overeating. Effectively, the best way to gain body size and bulk along with progressive loading is eating more than you're hungry for (more calories in than out) with focus on proteins and starchy complex carbohydrates. Then, there are enhancement drugs. The most known being anabolic steroids and other testosterone-boosting supplements.

NOTE: if the body can be strengthened and bulked up with progressive loading and increased calorie intake from carbohydrates, it's more than fair to understand that the same body can be strengthened and toned up without the bulk by confining resistance load and carbohydrates intake to the optimum. That's precisely what gTonnicks' The Sleekest Workout Program is about.

PART 3:
UNDERSTANDING THE SLEEKFIT EATING

"Strive for progress, not perfection"

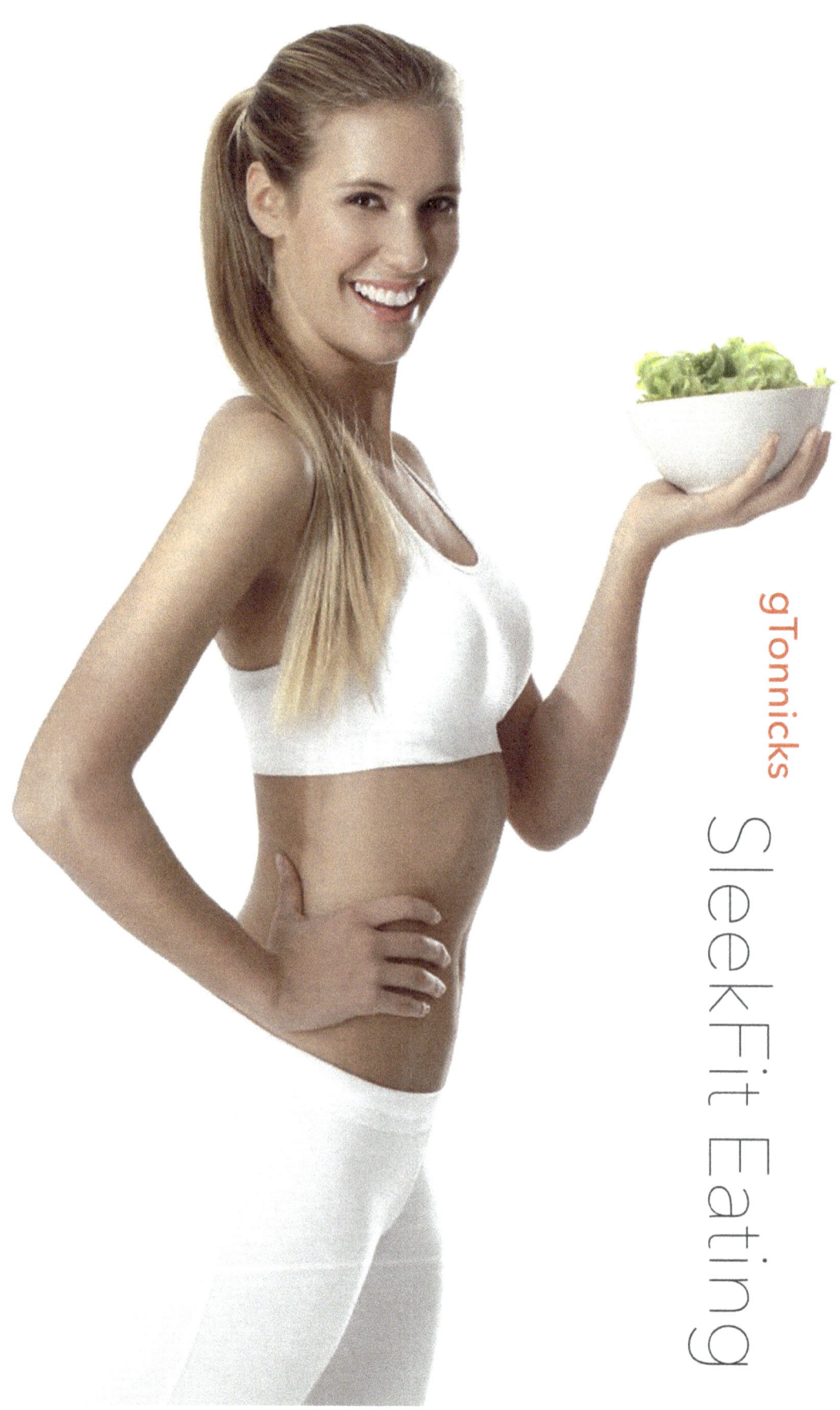

gTonnicks

SleekFit Eating

Part 3: Understanding the SleekFit Eating

All the workouts in the world will not yield the kind of physique you seek without proper eating. So, before anything, I would like you to understand the effects of food on the body, especially in conjunction with exercising.

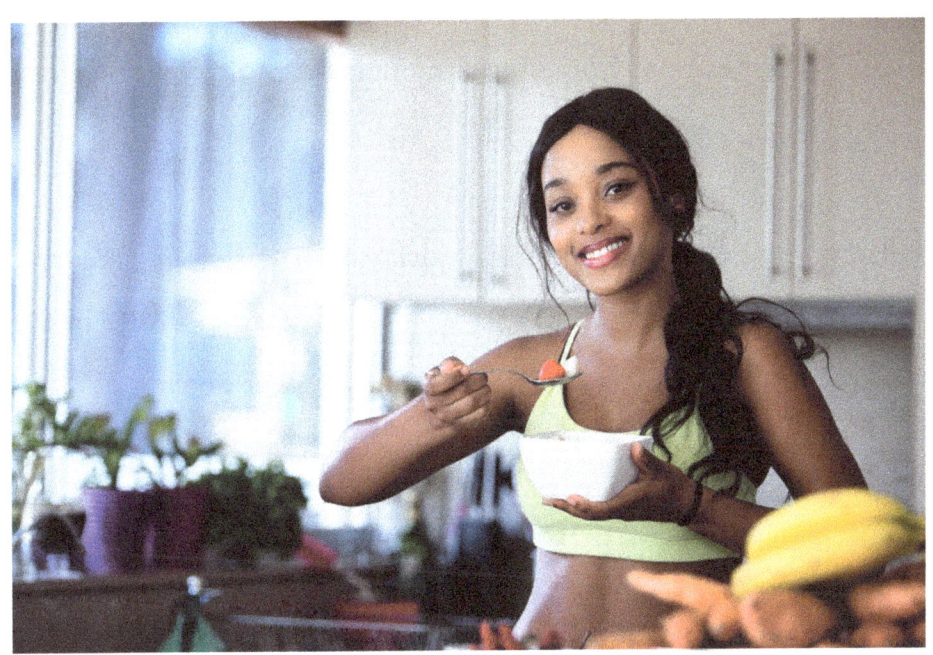

Starchy Complex Carbohydrates vs. Fibrous Complex Carbohydrates

A big part of the success of gTonnicks's The Sleekest Workout is based on the amounts of daily calories from the complex carbohydrates – the "good carbs" – you consume. As mentioned earlier, complex carbohydrates come in two forms: starchy carbohydrates and fibrous carbohydrates. For the purpose of gTonnicks' The Sleekest Workout program, the amount of starchy vs. fibrous carbohydrates depends on body genetic types.

That is, in general rules:

• If you aim to gain lean weight (ectomorph), you should have higher amounts of starchy complex carbohydrates.

• On the other hand, if you're an endomorph you likely want to lose weight. Therefore, you should have more amount of your calories from fibrous complex carbohydrates rather than from the starchy ones.

• If you have a mesomorph body type, you might just want to maintain and lean out, or only add a few pounds of lean (muscles) weight. Either way, it's best to keep a ratio of 50/50 to 75/25 of starches over fibers depending on your goals.

Keep It Simple and Consistent

Simplicity is the name of the game when it comes to SleekFit Eating. Below are the lists of foods in each category. Select the foods to eat from each category. Stick to the same selection week in week out for the entire program cycle (8 -12 weeks) with occasional substitutes. But the main foods should remain essentially the same. It makes it easier to prepare and keep up with. For many years I've had the same breakfast every day of the week: Steel-cut Oatmeal mixed with yogurt, mixed nuts, and whey protein altogether. On Sundays I make myself an egg omellette with slices of toasted whole grain bread since I'm off on those days and consequently have more time. It worked perfectly.

Timing is everything

Even though, the complex carbohydrates are the "good carbs", the consumption of them must be restricted to appropriated amounts daily. Those amounts vary among individuals based on each person's current bodyweight, physical activities, gender, fitness goals, and other factors like bio-chemical individualities or body genetics. Regardless of any amount of complex carbohydrates you take, it's crucial that you take it at the right time keeping in mind that it's the primary fuel for the body. I suggest having the biggest amount of your complex carbohydrates as part of first meal (breakfast) when you wake up and/or a certain amount of it about an hour before your gTonnicks' The Sleekest Workout session, and within 45 minutes after your gTonnicks' The Sleekest Workout session.

Watch the Starchy Carbs!

The starchy carbs are the ones I considered 'heavy" and substantial in nature. They're flour-based which gives them a high concentration of calories from glycogen (sugar) in them, which means they can be converted to fat relatively. It's so easy to consume too much of them because they taste good and are very satisfying. Example of starchy carbs are beans, rice, pasta, bread, and potatoes or anything of that nature. Unless you are under 30 years old with a high ectomorph) metabolism or very active (4 hours or more of training) athlete, it would be difficult stay lean with starchy carbs occupying most of calorie intake. For that reason, the fibrous carbohydrates are the prime choice over the starchy ones for your body fuel. Moreover, fibrous are loaded with vitamins and antioxidants (cleansing) against the free radicals. The free radicals are byproducts of fats and are known to intoxicate the body cells.

However, starchy complex carbohydrates intake before your workout provides fuel that helps sustain your efforts. Taking it after your workout helps replenish your body and actually allows you to burn fat throughout the rest of the day.

ALWAYS MIX YOUR CARBOHYDRATES WITH PROTEINS, ESPECIALLY AFTER A WORKOUT SESSION FOR BETTER ASSIMILATION OF PROTEINS.

The sweet poison:

We know now that all carbohydrates (complex, fibrous, or simple) get converted into sugar as necessary fuel for the body. However, there are refined food - through manufacturing process and other methods of extraction – are just downright dangerous for your health and fitness. They include sweeteners and others. See below for the effects of those sugars on your body:

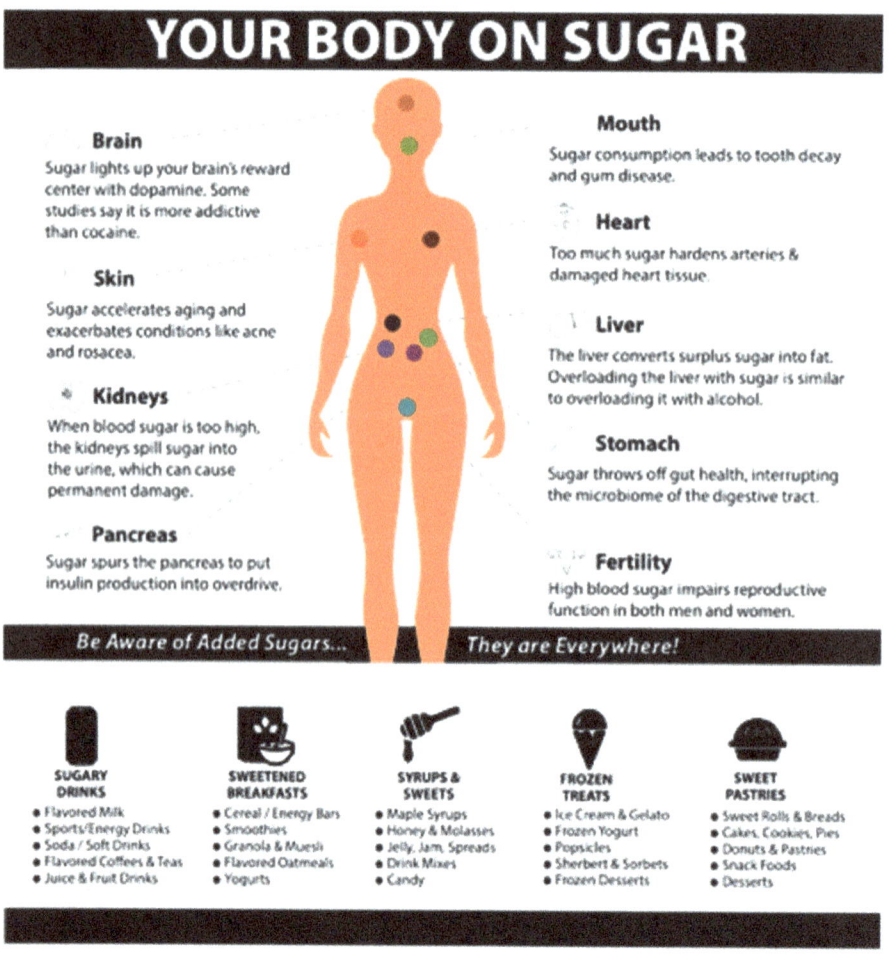

YOUR BODY ON SUGAR

Brain
Sugar lights up your brain's reward center with dopamine. Some studies say it is more addictive than cocaine.

Skin
Sugar accelerates aging and exacerbates conditions like acne and rosacea.

Kidneys
When blood sugar is too high, the kidneys spill sugar into the urine, which can cause permanent damage.

Pancreas
Sugar spurs the pancreas to put insulin production into overdrive.

Mouth
Sugar consumption leads to tooth decay and gum disease.

Heart
Too much sugar hardens arteries & damaged heart tissue.

Liver
The liver converts surplus sugar into fat. Overloading the liver with sugar is similar to overloading it with alcohol.

Stomach
Sugar throws off gut health, interrupting the microbiome of the digestive tract.

Fertility
High blood sugar impairs reproductive function in both men and women.

Be Aware of Added Sugars...   *They are Everywhere!*

SUGARY DRINKS
- Flavored Milk
- Sports/Energy Drinks
- Soda / Soft Drinks
- Flavored Coffees & Teas
- Juice & Fruit Drinks

SWEETENED BREAKFASTS
- Cereal / Energy Bars
- Smoothies
- Granola & Muesli
- Flavored Oatmeals
- Yogurts

SYRUPS & SWEETS
- Maple Syrups
- Honey & Molasses
- Jelly, Jam, Spreads
- Drink Mixes
- Candy

FROZEN TREATS
- Ice Cream & Gelato
- Frozen Yogurt
- Popsicles
- Sherbert & Sorbets
- Frozen Desserts

SWEET PASTRIES
- Sweet Rolls & Breads
- Cakes, Cookies, Pies
- Donuts & Pastries
- Snack Foods
- Desserts

ALSO:

1. Have breakfast as soon as you can after waking up. It boots up your metabolism.

2. Eat about every 2 and ½ hours to 3 hours between meals to maintain
a balanced blood sugar level.

3. Eat protein first, then fibrous (veggie or fruits) complex carbs, before the starchy complex carbs
to help control the amount of those starches.

4. Drink at least 8 oz. of water every hour.

5. Keep your complex carbohydrate intake down to the daily amount as recommended in this book
or by your nutritionist or registered dietitian.

6. See the list of foods provided to you for your selection of foods.

7. Pick a "cheat day" when you may indulge yourself with a 'not-so-healthy" food or drink. Just do
it moderately.

PART 4:
SETTING YOURSELF UP FOR SUCCESS

"Remember, if you don't know where you are going, any road will take you there."

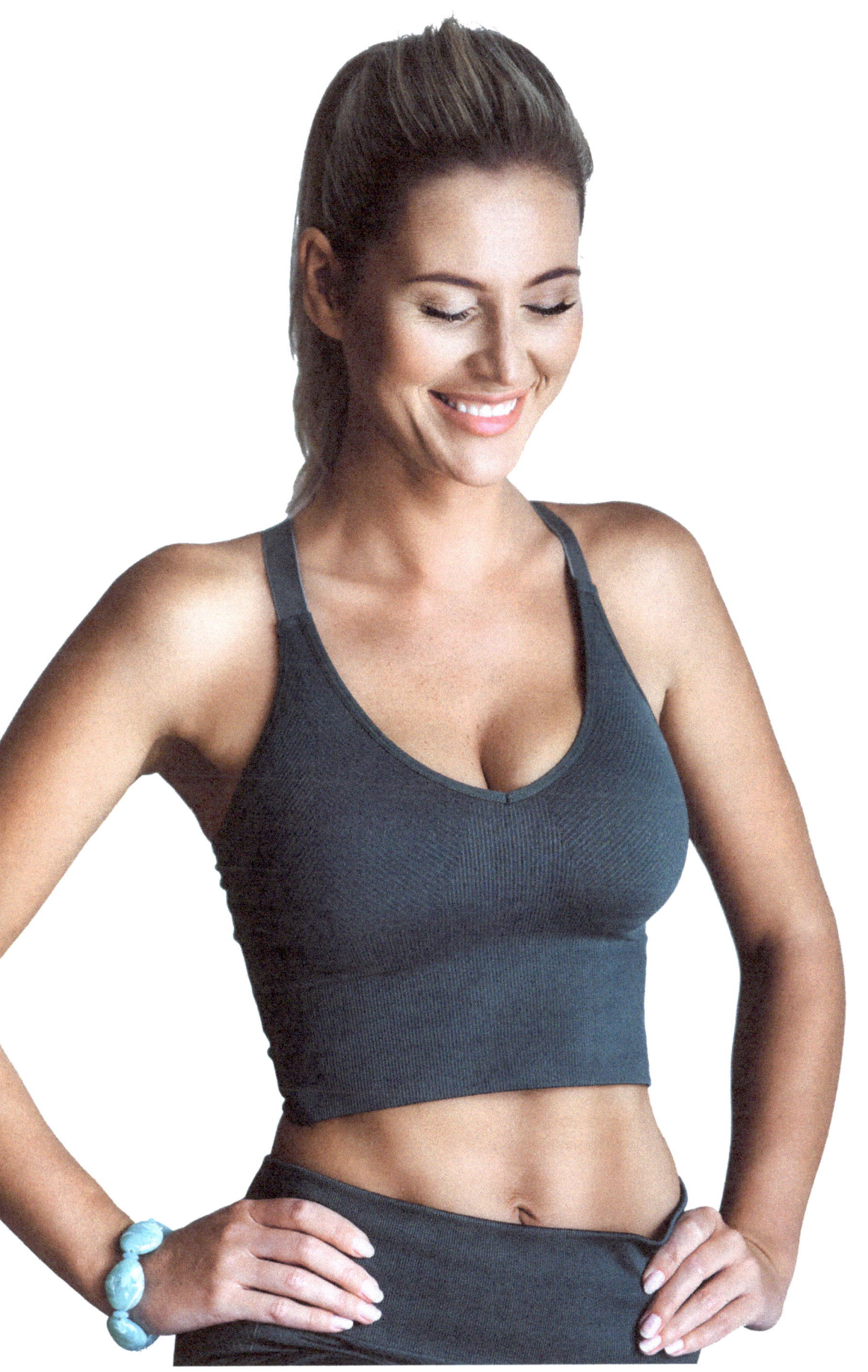

Part 4: Setting Yourself Up for Success

Prepare. Commit. Succeed.

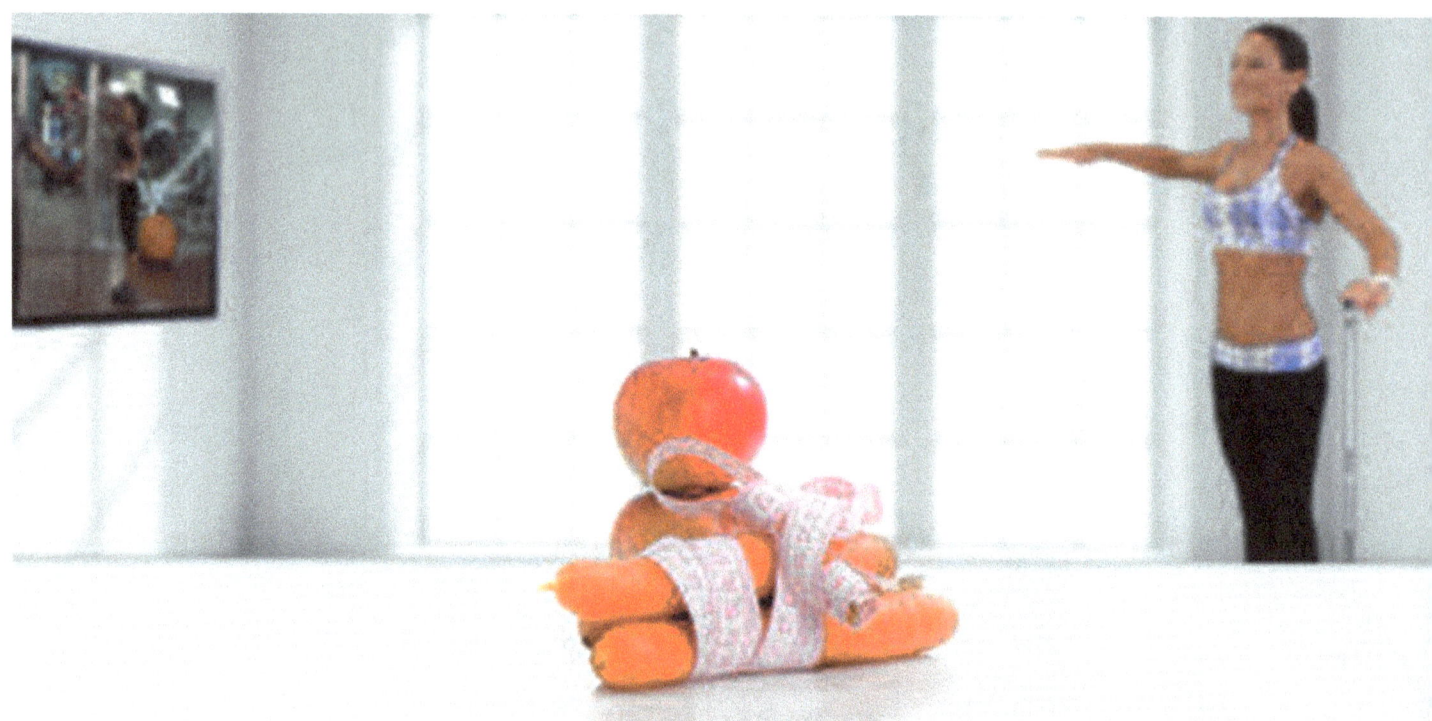

Calculating your estimated energy requirements (EER) based on you goal (gain/loss/maintain)? Figuring out how many calories a day you need to lose weight, maintain your weight or gain weight really isn't too hard. But, if you don't put a little time in figuring it out and adjusting your lifestyle to accommodate it, you will never reach your goals. There are a few reliable formulas out there namely, the Mifflin-St Jeor equation, the Katch McCardle formula, and the Cunningham one that you can try for yourself and compare with the one I'm giving you below. I've done the same and the numbers came darn close. With this formula you can easily track where you are and what you need to do daily to reach your goals.

"Remember, if you don't know where you are going, any road will take you there."

Step 1:

Take current body weight in pounds (lbs.) and multiply by 11.

Example: 139 lbs. x 11 = 1,529 calories.

This is what you need to just keep what you have, without moving. However, you do move. So, you have to then calculate your metabolic factors into this.

Step 2:

Estimate your metabolic factor according to the table below. But, first some mental refreshment on the 3 body (genetic) types descriptions, including your age to help you determine where you might fit in:

- **Mesomorph (slow metabolism):** You basically look at food and you seem to put on pounds. It's just difficult to lose weight and easy to gain it.

- **Endomorph (moderate metabolism):** You can gain weight if you try. You can lose weight if you try. You really don't have trouble losing weight depending on what you want to do.

- **Ectomorph (fast metabolism):** You are the skinny person who can eat *ANYTHING* and it makes no difference. Gaining weight is difficult. Losing weight can happen overnight. Just by watching television you seem to shed pounds.

Metabolic Percentage

Under 30 years old:

| Slow (endomorph) | Moderate (mesomorph) | Fast (ectomorph) |
| Metabolism- 30% | Metabolism- 40% | Metabolism- 50% |

30 - 40 years old:

| Slow (endomorph) | Moderate (mesomorph) | Fast (ectomorph) |
| Metabolism- 25% | Metabolism- 35% | Metabolism- 45% |

Over 40 years old:

| Slow (endomorph) | Moderate (mesomorph) | Fast (ectomorph) |
| Metabolism- 20% | Metabolism- 30% | Metabolism- 40% |

Example of a mesomorph between 30 and 40 years of age: 1529 calories x 35% = 535.15

Step 3:

Put it together. 1529 + 535.15 = 2064.15 calories.

You need 2064.15 calories to maintain your current weight with your current activities. This is called your Basal Metabolic Rate (BMR) how many calories your body burns daily without exercising. It's not 100% accurate (what is) but it's pretty good as I tried personally. You might need to adjust your metabolic factor when you start gTonnicks' The Sleekest Workout program. So, if you have a moderate metabolism and move to Phase 2 of gTonnicks' The Sleekest Workout for example, it might make more sense to put yourself in the fast metabolism category since you burn a lot more calories.

Step 4:

Now change the above with about 500 calories every day to reach your goals!

- Lose Weight: I would take 2064.15 – 500 = 1565.15

• Maintain Weight: I would just leave it at 2064.15 and continue what I was doing in my activities

- Gain Weight: I would take 2064.15 + 500 = 2564.15

NOTE: *500 calories a day is just a general term everybody uses to say that adding this amount is within safe limits. Eat too much, and you end up storing fat. Cut too many calories and your body just goes into starvation mode and ends up retaining more fat. 500 is a safe, recommended guideline.*

Necessary Measurements

Calories from Carbohydrates: Most nutritionists and registered dietitians recommend 45 percent to 65 percent of carbohydrate intake or about 130 grams a day. In association with gTonnicks' The Sleekest Workout program, I would suggest that you take 4 to 7 grams a day per kilogram of your bodyweight. That is 4 to 7g/kg/BW/day with the lower end of your carbohydrate intake (4 grams) being on the alternate day (see workout schedule) of the program.

So, using the 139 lbs. body weight again as an example:

139 lbs. = 63.05 kilograms. That's 252.2 grams to 441.35 grams of carbohydrates a day, which yield 1,008.80 to 1,765.40 calories daily just from carbohydrates.

Complex (starchy) Carbohydrates Intake

The following categories of recommended calorie intake are established based on your current body weight, desired weight, and the amount of complex carbohydrates (starches) and protein you need.

As a female of:

115 – 129 lbs. bodyweight take 60 – 80 g (240 – 320 calories) of starchy carbohydrates.

130 – 149 lbs. bodyweight take 80 - 120 g (240 – 480 calories) of starchy carbohydrates.

150 - 200 lbs. bodyweight take 120 - 170 g (520 – 680 calories) of starchy carbohydrates.

Over 200 lbs. bodyweight take 170 - 200 g (680 – 800 calories) of starchy carbohydrates.

Important Notice:

The remaining of your calorie intake shall come from the fruits, vegetable (fibrous carbohydrates), and proteins featured in the Food List.

Vegetable (fibrous carbohydrates) Intake

You may have as much as fibrous carbohydrates as desired or as suggested.

See the list of veggies sources and recommended amounts on the SleekFit!™ diet food list.

TIPS:

• Now, make sure that about 25 percent of those calories from carbohydrates come from the fibrous (green, leafy, colorful veggies and whole fruits) carbohydrates and the remaining from starchy carbohydrates.

• limit your fruit intake to 3 or 4 servings daily and spread throughout the day. Have them whole preferably.

• If you're trying to lose weight, make it about 50/50 percent of the fibrous and starches carbohydrates on workout day of gTonnicks' The Sleekest Workout program and 75/25 percent of the fibrous and starches carbohydrates on the alternate days of the program.

• If you're trying to gain lean bodyweight (muscles), up your calorie intake from starches up to the 7 grams per bodyweight in kilograms per day with the only 25 percent of it coming from the fibrous carbohydrates even on your alternate day of the workout schedule.

Calories from Proteins

According the Recommended Dietary Allowance (RDA), the general protein requirement for a sedentary person is 0.8 g/kg BW/day. However, this requirement can be elevated to meet the need of gTonnicks' The Sleekest Workout program. So, I would suggest 1.2 grams to 2.2 grams (g/kg BW/day) daily. So, that's 75.66 grams to 138.71 grams daily for the 139 lbs. bodyweight example.

PROTEIN GRAM CALCULATOR

MEATS	CHICKEN	EGGS	FISH	SHELLFISH	CHEESE
3.5 ounces is about the size of a deck card and equals 25-30 g	About 1 breast or 2 drumsticks equals 25-30 g	1 large egg equals 6 grams	3 ounces fresh or frozen equals 20-25 g.	3 ounces of lobster meat 12 lg. Shrimp 6 lg. Scallops 9 sm. Oysters equals 10-15 g	Hard: equals 6-7 g. per ounce. Soft: Equals 3-4 g per ounce

The acceptable micronutrient range for fat intake is 20 to 35 percent of energy. The fat requirements for sedentary individuals and athletes are similar, but slightly higher for athletes. Consuming adequate amounts of fat is required for optimal health, maintenance of energy balance, optimal intake of essential fatty acids and fat-soluble vitamins, as well as replenishing intramuscular triglyceride stores. It's not recommended to take less than 15 to 20%. Example: So, of the 2064.15 calorie requirements, 412.83 to 722.45 calories would come from the "good fats".

NOW, THROW IT ALL OUT OF THE WINDOW!

It might sound crazy for me to say that after just emphasizing the importance of knowing how much calories or energy intake you need, but those "necessary" measurements are just to be used as an initial reference. Don't get yourself boggle down to counting calories every time or ever after that. Once you measure foods, you will have a good idea how much (portion size) is what. Use portion sizes instead, which those initial "necessary" measurements help you determine. Then make those portion sizes more or less base on how you feel energy wise after you eat. It will take a few days to get it right and make it an almost mindless game without stress. Your body and the way you feel physically are your best indicators, thus making you your own expert of your body needs to stay fit.

It will take you about 2 weeks to totally understand and implement the SleekFit! During this learning and application phase, you will get to appreciate how simple and easy it is to follow. After the initial first weeks, you wouldn't even need to calculate anything. You will only follow the portions as pre-determined, except for occasional adjustments as your body shape up nicely.

Phase 1: The First Two Weeks

What can you eat and what should you avoid in the crucial first two weeks? If you're looking to lose weight, you should get most of your calories from proteins (meat, fish, poultry, dairy, and other sources listed in the Food List) and from the fibrous complex carbohydrates. Avoid the starchy complex carbohydrates for now. You'll have a portion of protein about the size of the palm of your hand for breakfast, lunch, and dinner. Don't worry if you're a vegetarian or vegan; there's plenty for you to eat, too. Nor need you worry too much about how you cook (or don't cook your food) at this point. Preferably, sauté your protein in olive or canola oil or grill it. Preferred vegetable cooking methods are steaming, sautéing, or sir-frying in a wok. Don't deep-fry any food or overcook any vegetable. You may want to pick a "cheat day" to occasionally indulge yourself with a 'not-so-healthy" food or drink. Just do it moderately.

Phase 2: Carbs In!

You will now carefully introduce starchy carbohydrate into your diet. Refer to the Complex Carbohydrate Intake Table or consult with your registered dietitian or nutritionist to see which category you fit in for your recommended daily starchy carbohydrate amounts.

Phase 3: Longevity

Once you've reached your desired and healthy body weight and shape, you will want to maintain it. There is no going back, is there? So, you are now in the longevity phase for the rest of life. Below is an example of what your weekly eating plan might look like. Keep it in mind that the most important is to control the amount of complex carbohydrates you take daily while keeping your protein and lots of veggies in. Consult with your physician regularly.

CHOOSING PROPER NUTRITION

Plate Method

The U.S. Department of Agriculture's ChooseMyPlate is one of the simplest methods for measuring out the right proportions of foods. Divide a 9-inch plate into four sections and fill one section with protein, one with non-starchy vegetables, one with fruit or another non-starchy vegetable and one with grains or starchy vegetables. Add an 8-ounce glass of milk or another serving of dairy for a complete meal.

Measuring

Another method is to use measuring cups and a food scale. The numbers of servings from each food group depend on age, gender and activity level. However, most adults should consume 1 1/2 to 2 cups of fruit, 2 to 3 cups of vegetables, 5 to 8 ounces of grains, 5 to 6 1/2 ounces of protein foods and 3 cups of dairy. Women and less active people should aim for the lower amount, and men and more active people may need the higher amount.

Estimation

It isn't always possible to weigh or measure your food to get the proper proportions, and not everyone wants to go to this trouble. You can estimate how many servings you are consuming by comparing your food to common items. For example, 1 ounce of cheese is about the same size as four dice, 3 ounces of meat is about the same size as a deck of cards or your palm and a cup is about the size of a woman's fist.

Considerations

Check nutrition labels to determine how large a serving is and how many servings are in a container; that way, you won't inadvertently eat multiple servings. Try to choose less energy-dense and more nutrient-dense items within each food group to get the most nutrition with the fewest calories. Opt for vegetables without high-fat sauces, whole grains over refined grains, along with low-fat dairy products and lean meats. One of the most significant ways to decrease empty calories is to include more vegetables in your meals.

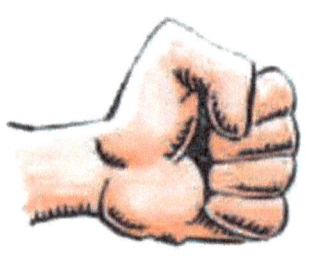 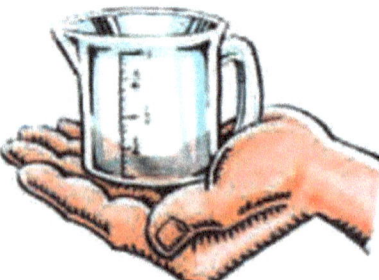

A fist or cupped hand = 1 cup

1 serving = 1/2 cup cereal, cooked pasta or rice
or 1 cup of raw, leafy green vegetables
or 1/2 cup of cooked or raw, chopped
vegetables or fruit

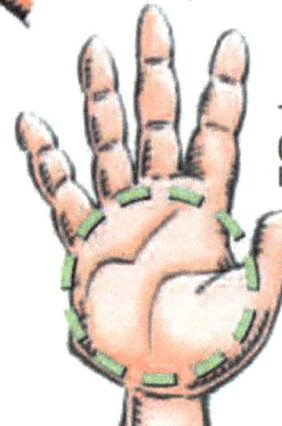

Palm = 3 oz. of meat

Two servings, or 6 oz., of lean meat
(poultry, fish, shellfish, beef) should
be a part of a daily diet. Measure
the right amount with your
palm. One palm size portion
equals 3 oz.,
or one serving.

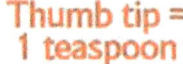

Thumb tip = 1 teaspoon

Keep high-fat foods, such as
peanut butter and mayonnaise,
at a minimum by measuring
the serving with your thumb.
One teaspoon is equal to the end
of your thumb, from the knuckle up.
Three teaspoons
equals 1 tablespoon.

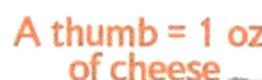

A thumb = 1 oz. of cheese

Consuming low-fat
cheese is a good
way to help you meet
the required servings
from the milk, yogurt
and cheese group.
1 1/2 - 2 oz. of low-fat
cheese counts as 1 of the 2-3
daily recommended servings.

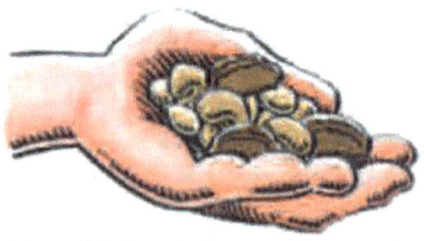

Handful = 1-2 oz. of snack food

Snacking can add up. Remember, 1 handful
equals 1 oz. of nuts and small candies. For chips
and pretzels, 2 handfuls equals 1 oz.

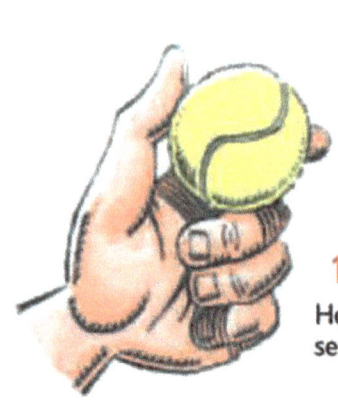

1 tennis ball = 1 serving of fruit

Healthy diets include 2-4
servings of fruit a day.

Your List of Foods

The following lists of foods are to go with your gTonnicks' The Sleekest Workout program for best results. They are selected based on their glycemic index (GI) and glycemic load (GL) among other qualities.

Complex Starchy Carbohydrates

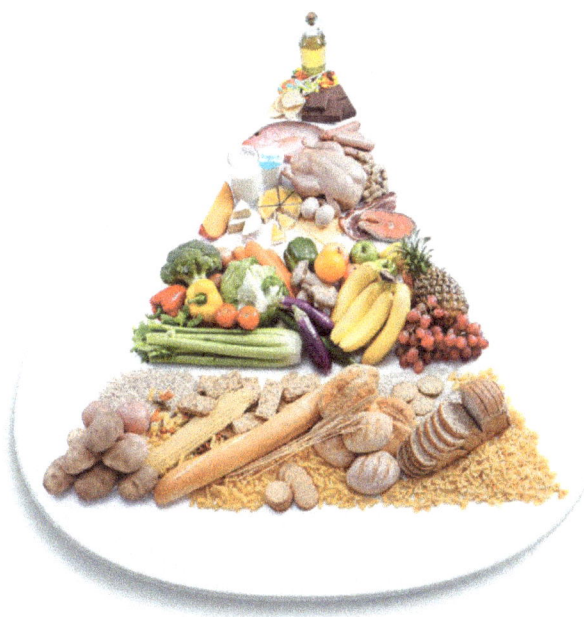

Have your carbohydrates fresh and natural, and at the right amount without added calories from sweets and other ingredients.

- Whole Grain Bread (gluten free if you're allergic)
- Rice (any type)
- Sweet Potato
- Red Potato
- Yam
- Oatmeal
- Beans
- Peas
- Pasta

Complex Fibrous Carbohydrates (greens)

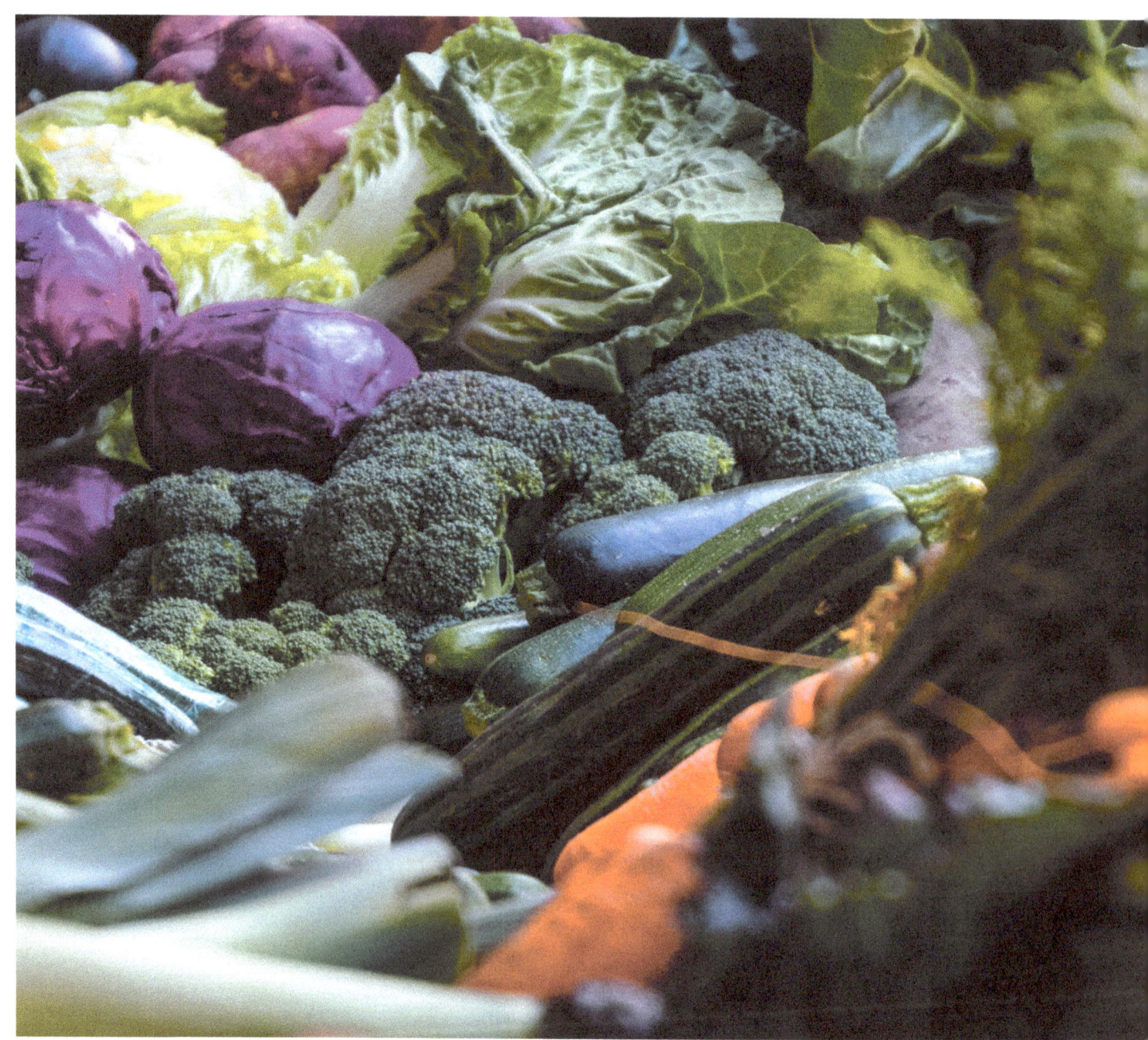

• **Unlimited** - You can eat unlimited amounts of the following veggies

(add to salads or eat raw as a snack):

Celery
Chives
Cucumbers
Jicana
Lettuce
Mushrooms
Olives
Onion (Raw 2-3 rings)
Parsley
Peppers (All Types)
Salad mixed

• **Limited** - You can eat limited amounts of the following veggies:

Artichokes
Asparagus (8 spears)
Bean Sprouts
Broccoli
Brussels sprouts
Cabbage
Carrots Celery
Cauliflower
Eggplant
Garlic
Green beans
Greens (collard, turnip, mustard, beet, kale, etc.)
Kohlrabi
Leeks
Mushrooms
Pea pods
Spinach
Summer Squash
Tomato
Water chestnuts
Yellow crook-neck
Zucchini
Zucchini/squash,

Complex Fibrous Carbohydrates (fruits)

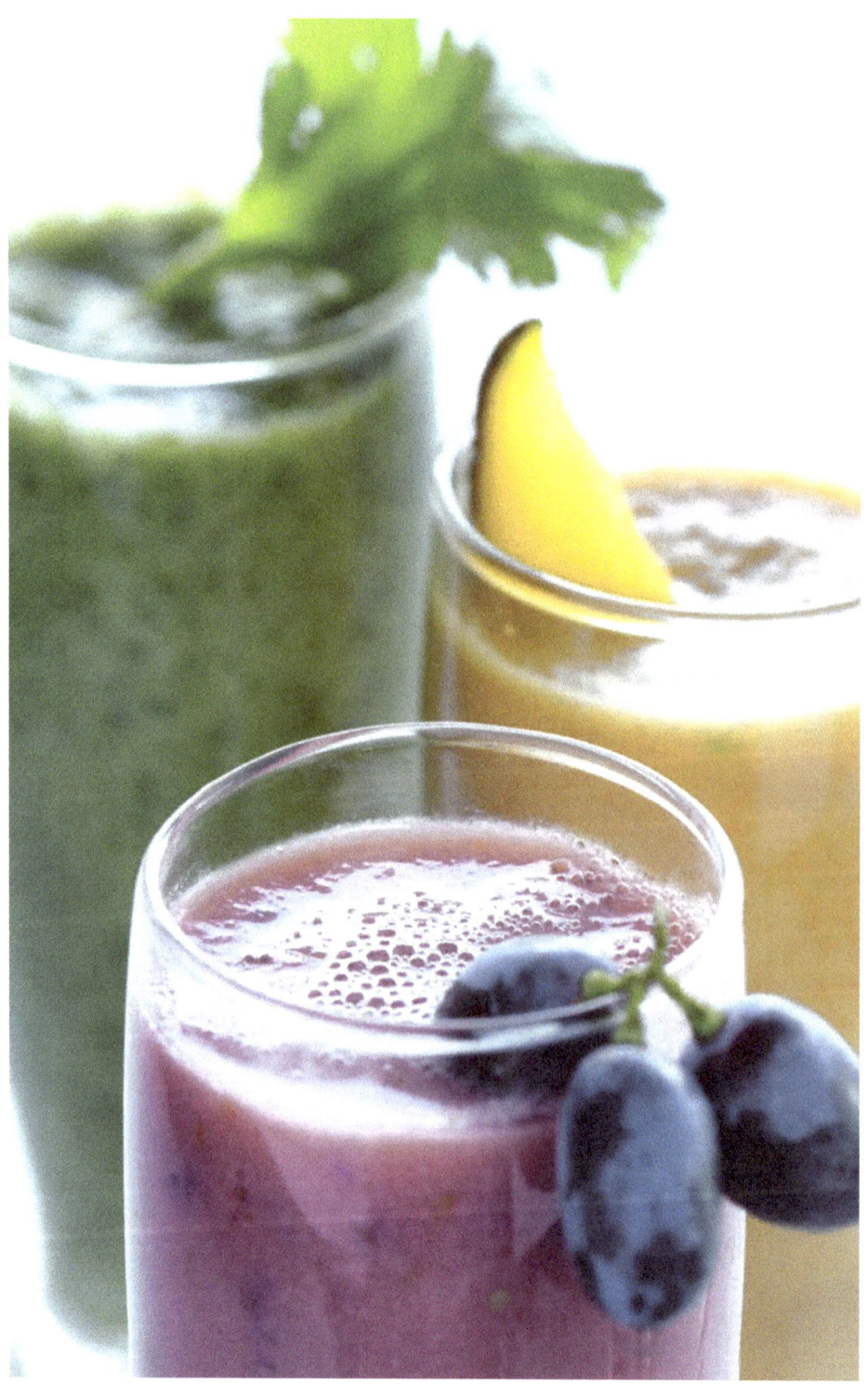

Have one fruit or serving

up to 3 times daily:

Apples
Apricots
Avocados
Bananas (green tip)
Berries (all kinds)
Cantaloupe
Grapefruit
Grapes
Guava
Kiwi
Mango
Nectarines
Oranges
Peaches
Pears
Pears
Plums

Carbohydrate Nutritional Information

Food	Amount	Carbs	Calories	Protein
Banana	Medium 8"	26.70 g	105	1.20 g
Orange	Medium	15 g	62	1.2 g
Apple	Medium (with peel)	21 g	81	0.3 g
Bread (Whole wheat)	1 slice	13 g	70	3 g
Bread (Rye, 7 grain)	1 slice	18 g	90	2.5 g
Brown Rice	1 cup	49 g	232	5 g
Kidney Bean (boiled)	1 cup	39 g `	218	16 g
Lentil (boiled)	1 cup	40 g	230	18 g
Oatmeal (uncooked)	1 cup	56 g	297	13 g
Yam (baked/boiled)	1 cup	33 g	158	2 g
Sweet Potato (raw)	1	26 g	112	2 g
Green Beans (string boiled/drained)	5 ounces	11 g	50	3 g
Black Beans (boiled)	1 cup	40.78 g	227.04	15 g
Peanut Butter	1 tsp	3.50 g	95	4 g
Potato	5 ounces	84 g	155	3.25 g
Corn Tortilla	1 each	9 g	45	1 g

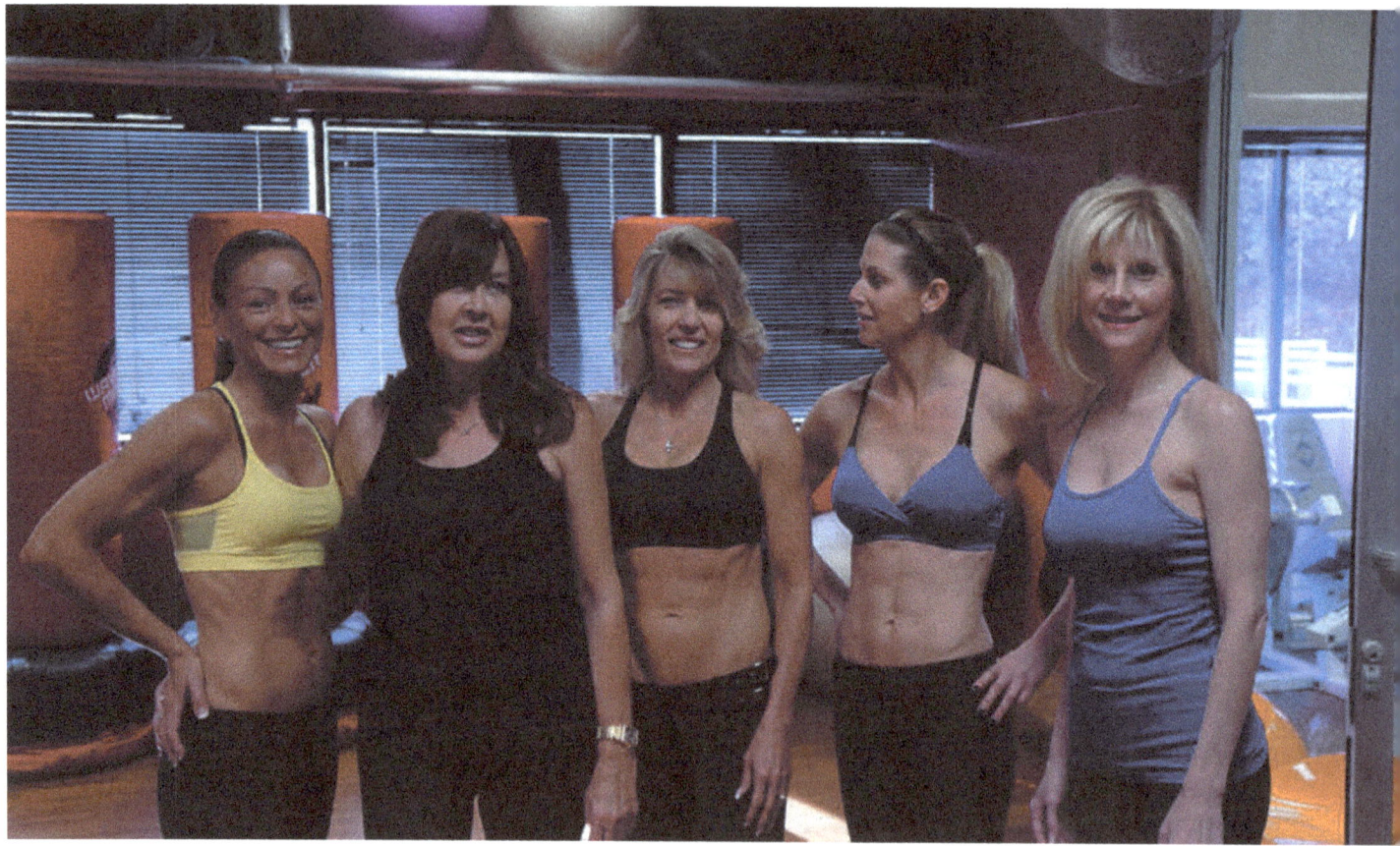

PROTEINS: Prepare your protein dishes any way you want except breaded.

FRESH MEATS	POULTRY	SHELLFISH	EGGS	FISH
Beef	Chicken	Shrimp	Scrambled	All kinds
Pork	Turkey	Lobster	Over-easy	2-3 servings
Lamb	Duck	Oysters	Hard-boiled	Recommended:
Bacon*	Quail	Clams	Poached	deep sea, cold-water fish
Sausage*	Cornish hen	Mussel	Deviled	e.g. salmon or tuna
*Bacon and sausage are	Allowed but look for brands	Without nitrates or nitrites and	No sugars. NO processed like	meats as hot dog or bologna

*bacon/sausage is allowed but brands without nitrates,
NO sugars or processed meats (hot dogs or bologna.)

Snack Foods
Recommended while you follow gTonnicks' The Sleekest Workout program:

Almonds
Berries
Chicken or meat
Cottage cheese
Dry Turkey
Oranges
Peanuts
Plain yogurt
Pumpkin seeds

Garnishes (seasoning):
Grated cheese
Chopped hardboiled egg
Crumbled bacon
(No "fake" bits.)

Life quality and longevity

Once you've reached your desired and healthy body weight and shape, you will want to maintain it. There is no going back, is there? So, you are now in the longevity phase for the rest of life. Do your best to stick to following recommendations as part of food intake:

Dairy and Eggs: Cheese Cottage, Cheese, Ricotta cheese, Eggs, Egg substitute, Egg whites, Light margarine, Milk, Sour cream, Yogurt.

Condiments: Honey, Horseradish, Low-fat dressing, Mustard/Mayo** Salsa/Vinegars

Cereals: Cheerios, Oatmeal, Raisin Bran, Shredded wheat, Wheat Chex, Any whole.

Staples: Peanut butter, Almonds, Walnuts, Brown rice, White rice, Bulgur, Couscous, Wheat germ, Lentils, Dry beans, Dry split peas, Garlic powder, Imitation butter, Cajun spices, Mexican spices, Spices & Flavoring, Vanilla, S/F sweetener, Canola oil, Cooking oil, Cooking spray, Raisins, Dried Fruit, Flaxseeds.

Canned Goods: Tuna, Salmon, Black beans, Kidney beans, Lima beans, Garbanzo beans, Peas, Spinach, Tomatoes, Soup, Broth, Pineapple, Peaches, Pears, Applesauce*, Tomato sauce

Protein source: Chicken breast, Pre-cooked chicken strips, Beef (pot roast), Round steak, Pork tenderloin, Lean ground beef, Lean ground turkey, Salmon***, Halibut***, Orange Roughy***, Shark*** Red snapper, Scallops, Venison, Canadian-bacon, Leg of lamb, Lean ham, Lean deli meats, Tofu.

Pasta and sauce: Spaghetti, Macaroni, Noodles, Pasta sauce**

Beverages: Water, Coffee, Tea

*UNSWEETENED, **NON-FAT, ***FRESH PRODUCTS

Your meal schedule

Below is an example of what your daily eating plan might look like. Keep it in mind that the most important is to control the amount of complex carbohydrates you take daily while keeping your protein and lots of veggies in. Consult with your physician regularly.

Meal 1 (Breakfast)
- Complex Carbohydrates
- Protein
- Fruit (if recommended)

Meal 2 (mid-day)
- Healthy snack
- And/or Protein

Meal 3 (lunch)
- Lean protein food
- Large Green salad or mixed green veggies
- Fruit (if recommended)

Meal 4 (mid-afternoon)
- Healthy snack
- And/or Protein

Meal 5 (dinner)
- Lean protein food: steak, fish, poultry, or other.
- Green vegetables
- Fruit (if recommended)

Meal 6 (before bedtime)
- Healthy snack
- And/or Protein

The SleekFit Eating is one that we have used for years to guide clients, students and serious athletes alike. This meal plan is as non-restrictive and complex as possible, so it is very easy to follow and will get you results. Remember, Knowledge is Power! It is designed as a guide, so feel free to substitute with other foods you might like (as long as they are healthy and similar). One very important tip for success – find something that you like, something that tastes good to you and is easy to prepare. Good nutrition, like a good exercise program, should not be a chore. Rather something you look forward to doing. Try to select a variety of foods. It's more fun and you are more likely to stick with it. Also, just as important, stay in tune with your body. If you listen to your body you will know when "enough is enough." And when you can push it further without "breaking". gTonnicks' The Sleekest Workout requires just that as you will learn.

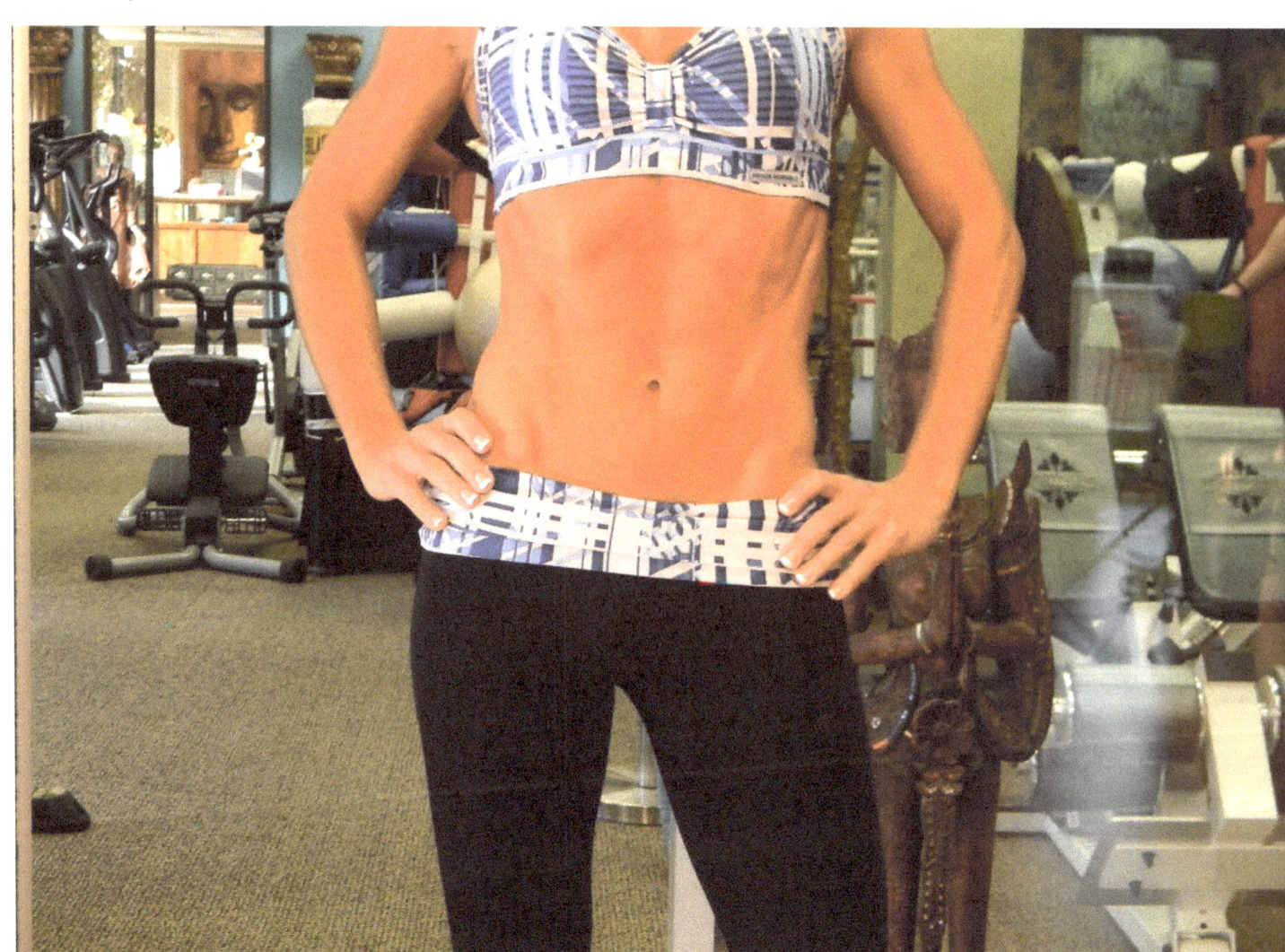

The Process:

• **Clear your refrigerator and your house of all bad foods.** Come on, you know what they are: potato chips, cookies, ice cream, cake, etc. These should be treats, not a part of your regular diet. Our rule of thumb is: "don't buy it and you won't eat it!" Or at least, don't buy enough to last a week.) Replace them with healthy, energizing foods.

• **Take your body measurements.**
You have to know where you are, to know where you want to be.

• **Start your workout and eating programs on a Monday.** It is always good to start at the beginning of the week. Plan to relax on the weekend, give your body a chance to recover and store up energy for the upcoming week. Rest is progress here.

• **Start with small goals.** If you desire to lose 40 pounds, set your initial goal at 2 pounds for the first two weeks. Aim to take inches off your waist area, before even thinking "six-pack" abs! You don't need it.

• **Plan your workouts.** If you plan your workouts within one hour from your mealtime, use a Meal Replacement Drink, or a healthy nutritional bar instead of a solid meal, which may weigh you down and possibly upset your stomach during your workout.

• **Decrease starches.** If you are planning to lose weight, you should decrease consumption of starches such as: like pasta, rice, potato, bread, and beans for lunch.

• **Increase starches.** On the other hand, if your goal is to add more lean weight, you should increase the consumption of starches such as: like pasta, rice, potato, bread, and beans for lunch.

In Summary

• Determine your body (or genetic) type. See descriptions of the three main body types to see where you best fit in.

• Determine your BMR. Follow the formula provided earlier to determine your basic calorie intakes

• Determine your EER

• Select your food Selection. Keep it simple and repetitive.

•Pick a start day

• Begin!

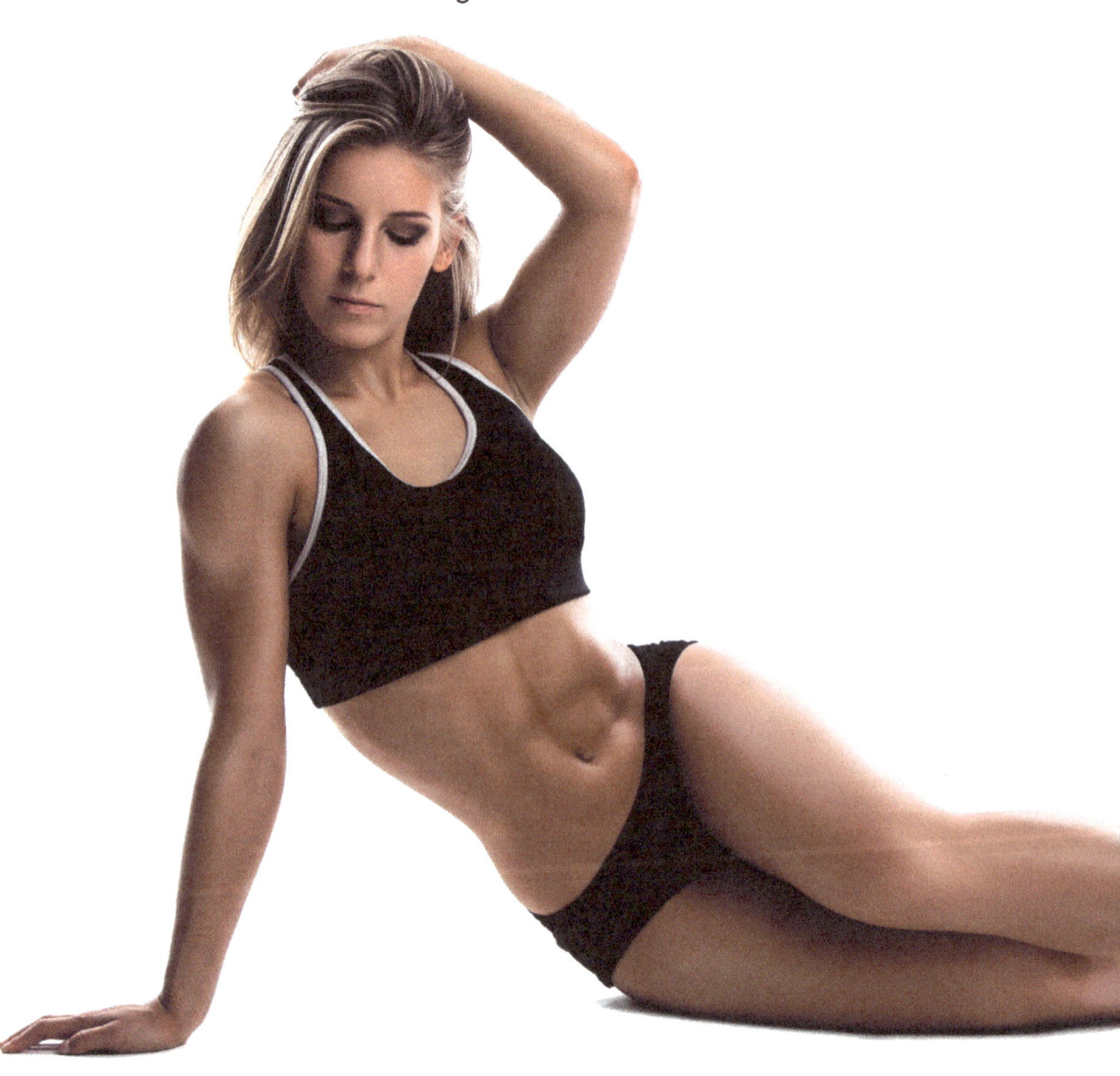

ADDENDUM

PART 5:
UNDERSTANDING FOOD & EXERCISING

"You only fail when
you stop trying"

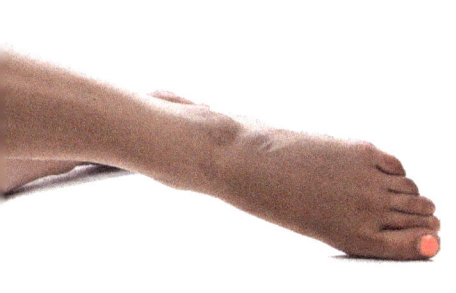

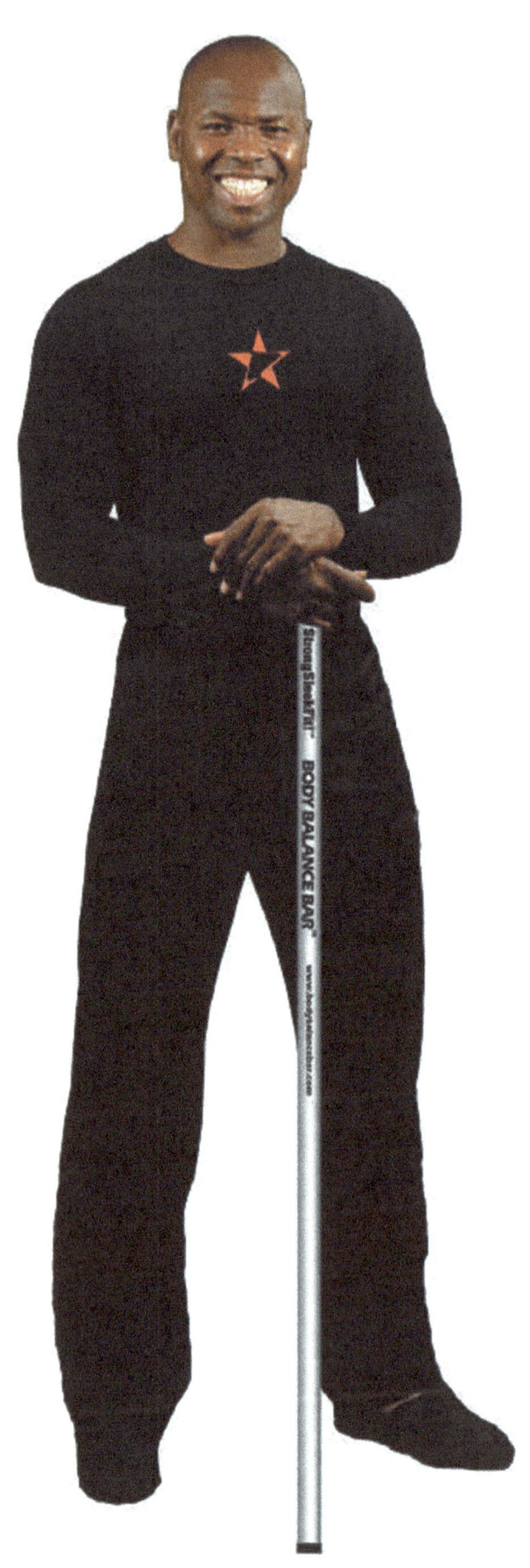

Part 5: Understanding Food & Exercising

Food is the biggest component under our control to regulate our body weight. However, it's usually the hardest component to change – because most nutritional programs are complex and quite restrictive, requiring you to alter and change your lifestyle in ways you can't maintain. These programs rarely work long-term, because you simply give them up and go back to your natural eating patterns. However, as many gTonnicks clients and students have learned over the years – "You may workout religiously — but you'll never achieve your fitness goals without proper eating habits." Healthy eating habits have to become a "natural part of your daily routine." Yes, you have to develop an eating "lifestyle" that you can maintain without any effort at all. It has to be practical, knowledge-based, and easy to implement. This guide seeks to give you, an "easy to follow, practical guide to daily nutrition."

Some of the information is elementary, but you have to "know why you are doing something," to really fully appreciate and get motivated to do it correctly. So, here are some the reasons why we all do need "good" eating habits:

• **Energy** – it's fuel for one of the most complex machines the world has ever known, the body!

• **Strength and Power** – an overlooked aspect of general health and fitness.

• **Lean Muscle** – the kind that most of us want – and lean muscles for better quality of life.

• **Decrease and Manage Body Fat** – without proper diet, you can exercise 4 hours a day, and never see the best results of your training.

• **Better Healing** – it has been proven that a good nutritional program will improve all body functions, aid in the healing and recovery of injuries, stimulate mental concentration, build and repair damaged tissues, speed recovery between workouts, and facilitate improved sleep and physical rest, and more.

Of course, no single food provides all the above benefits. The key is a good variety and balance of foods. Below are some of the things that affect your metabolism (how fast you burn food):

• Your current fitness level

• Your fitness goals

• The type activity and exercise you are currently performing

• Your current physical condition (illness, pregnancy, injury, out of shape, etc.)

• Your environment (hot or cold weather, dry or humid)

Here are four categories of foods and their functions you should become familiar with:

- Carbohydrates
- Proteins
- Fats
- Vitamins, Minerals, and Water

Each of the macronutrients – carbohydrates, fats, and proteins – plays an important role in fueling the body during an exercise session. The body stores these energy sources in various locations and releases them for use depending on the type of activity performed.

Carbohydrates generally come in two forms: sugars and starches. Sugars are often referred to as simple carbohydrates because your body can digest them quickly and easily. Simple carbohydrates are structurally known as monosaccharides. Three monosaccharides found in nature can be absorbed by humans: glucose, fructose, and galactose. Glucose is the predominant monosaccharide in nature and the basic bock of most other carbohydrates. Fructose is the sweetest of the monosaccharides and is found in varying levels in different types of fruits. Galactose is most often bound to glucose to form the disaccharide lactose, the principal sugar found in milk. Furthermore, monosaccharides can be bound together by a glycosidic bond to form disaccharides, oligosaccharides, or polysaccharides.

Now Understand This! The body NEEDS carbohydrates!

That's why people who make the mistake of going without carbohydrates for long periods of time, eventually crave them so badly. This craving often leads to over consumption of carbs and obvious results: you gain weight faster and even put on more weight than you had before! It's about balance and developing a sensible, healthy diet that you can maintain, especially if you're starting a rigorous exercise program, or if you're an athlete.

I remember almost a couple of decades ago, during Baywatch Television Series hit, the case of a young woman lifeguard who worked at the swim pool near my work gym. I noticed how much she had lost weight within weeks and looking amazing. I asked her how she was doing it. She told me she was following a recommendation by a doctor not to eat carb at all and only have animal proteins, including fats from cheese and plants. I remember warning her about the potential "backfire" of such diet with zero carbohydrate, but what's my word's worth against the one of a Doctor? She didn't follow my advice to put carbohydrates back in her food intake before her body starts "fighting back" and "forced" her to eat carbs. That's exactly what happened just a few weeks after. The poor girl. Not only she gained back all of what she had lost in bodyweight, but she also added much more on. So, much that she quit her lifeguard job out of embarrassment. What happened? My educated take is that her body craved carbohydrates so much that she inevitably couldn't help, but to start eating carbohydrates. And when she did, she couldn't stop. Her body wouldn't let her. Like an ultra-dry sponge denied of any fluid for a longtime, her body sucked up onto the carbs and wouldn't let go. Unfortunately, there are so many cases like this one.

Morale of the story: eat your carbs!

The myth: "fad" diets haven't given the general population the impression that carbohydrates are "bad' when it comes to weight control. The belief is that carbohydrates make people fat or gain weight. This is not true as well as high-quality, minimally processed carbohydrates are consumed in appropriate portion sizes. Although, all carbohydrates do get ultimately broken into glucose not all carbohydrates are created equal. Depending on a carbohydrate's glycemic index, extent of processing, and other foods consumed at the same time, the blood glucose response varies. Because there is no scale or formula that determines carbohydrate quality, many health experts use glycemic index (GI) and glycemic load (GL) as proxies.

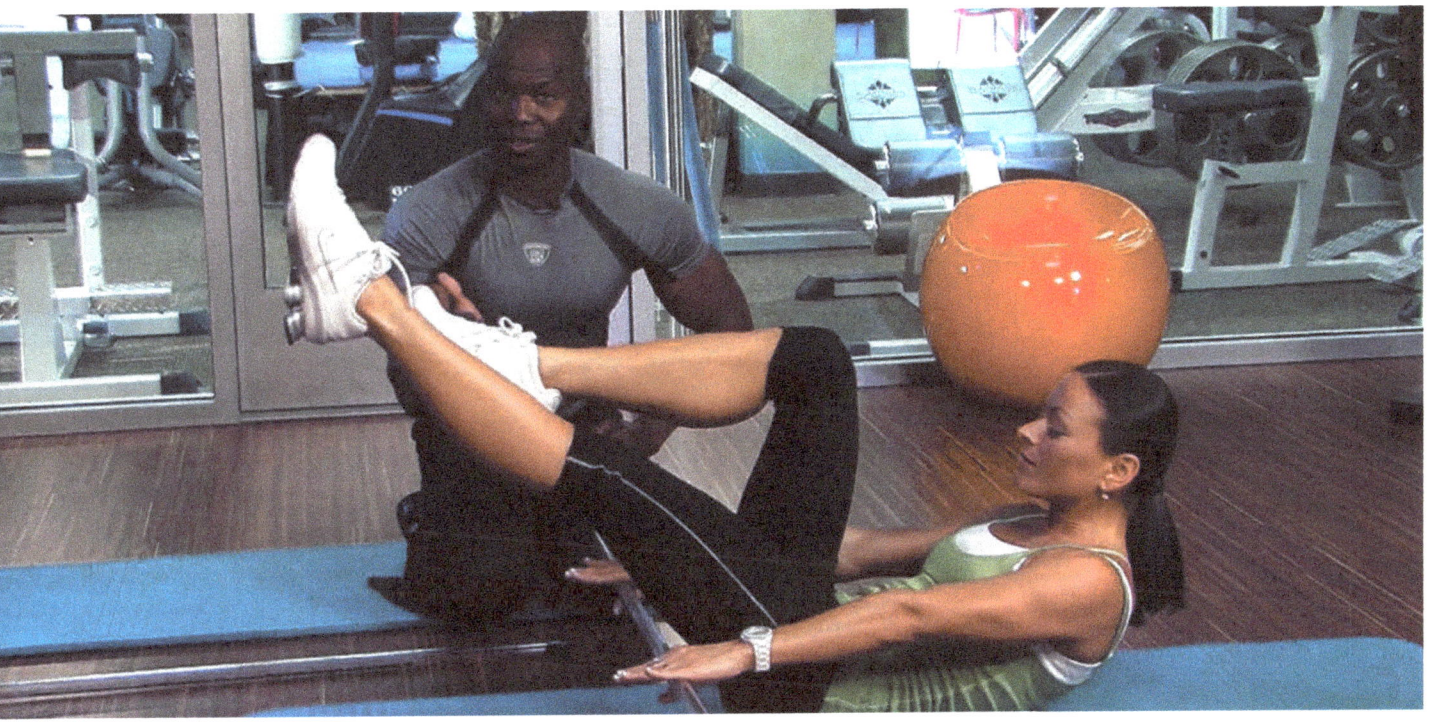

Glycemic Index and Glycemic Load

Glycemic index rings carbohydrates based on their blood glucose response. High-glycemic index foods enter the bloodstream rapidly, causing a large glucose spike. Then from 2 to 4 hours after consumption of high-glycemic index meal, residual effects from high insulin levels can cause a rapid drop in blood glucose and hypoglycemia.

On the other hand, low-glycemic index foods such as non-starchy vegetables, whole fruit, whole grains, and legumes are digested more slowly caused as smaller glucose increase and only a small boost blood insulin level. Highly processed, refined starches and sugar tend to have a higher glycemic index and have been associated with negative health consequences such as heart disease and diabetes.

While glycemic index is based on a reference form of carbohydrate, glycemic load (GL) accounts for portion sizes. In fact, a food with a high GI and a low GL therefore, can be a healthy choice. For example, while carrots have a high GI, they also have a low GL because to actually eat 50 grams of carrot, a person would need to eat 4 cups of the vegetable. Because the typical serving size is approximately one-half cup, the glycemic load is small.

Also, carbohydrate-containing foods that are also moderate to high in fat or protein, fiber, and all the nutrients and that are minimally processed may have a high glycemic index but a low glycemic load. Furthermore, Foods with a low glycemic load are commonly nutrient dense, meaning they provide more nutrients per calorie.

After being consumed, all carbohydrates are eventually digested to monosaccharides and absorbed into the bloodstream. The cells in the body use the monosaccharide form of glucose for energy. The other two monosaccharides, fructose and galactose, must be converted to glucose to be used by the cells as energy. Simple carbohydrates can also be a result of a highly manufacturing process. Starchy carbohydrates are referred to as complex carbohydrates because these carbohydrates take longer to be digested. Complex carbohydrates are structurally composed of oligosaccharides and polysaccharides.

Oligosaccharide is a chain of approximately three to ten simple sugars. They help relieve constipation, improve triglyceride (fat deposit) levels, and decrease production of foul-smelling digestive product.

Polysaccharides can consist of hundreds of monosaccharides bound together. They are three categories of polysaccharides: starch, fiber, and glycogen. Plants such as different grains and vegetables make starch, which is an energy source for the plant itself and provides carbohydrates for animals that consume the plant.

While other carbohydrates contain 4 calories per gram, fiber probably contributes about 1.3 to 2.5 calories per gram. They have no cholesterol and are low in calories and fat, and contain a variety of essential vitamins and minerals, including vitamins A, C and E, folate and potassium. The greener and darker the fibrous complex carbohydrates are, the more nutritious they are known to be. Additionally, the fibrous carbohydrates are loaded with antioxidants (cleansing elements) and fibers, which slow down digestion and facilitate food absorption and bowl movement. They are two kinds of fibers: soluble (dissolve in water) and non-soluble (doesn't dissolve in water). Dietary Fiber occupies a big portion of your complex carbohydrate intake in this program because of its health benefits, including digestion.

Because all those benefits attributed to the fibrous complex carbohydrates, including low calorie (2.2 to 2.8 calories per gram) most your calorie intake should derive from them as part of your gTonnicks' The Sleekest Workout program for a strong, sleek, and fit you.

Carbohydrates as Fuel

Carbohydrates serves as the body's preferred energy source and help to fend off the fatigue and exhaustion that threatens the end of a prolonged workout. Carbohydrates are ideally suited to provide fuel for the metabolic functions, including that of the brain. Do you know that the brain, which weighs approximately three pounds consumes about 20 percent of the body's calories? Carbohydrates occupies a major role in the production of adenosine triphosphate (ATP), which is a chemical compound required for all cellular work. Importantly, carbohydrates are the only macronutrient whose stored energy generates ATP anaerobically. This is crucial during maximal exercise such as gTonnicks's The Sleekest Workout that requires rapid energy release above levels supplied by aerobic metabolism.

This is worth repeating this because it is very important:

DO NOT FORCE YOUR BODY TO USE PROTEIN FOR FUEL
BY DEPRIVING IT OF CARBOHYDRATES!

Remember the story about the lifeguard. Your body is a complex engine, with a memory, if you deprive your body of carbohydrates for too long, you will eventually CRAVE them, and upon resumed consumption, your body will seek to rapidly increase your "fat stores" because you have told it that you can't provide a reliable day source for it to draw upon. Thus, people who come off of carbohydrate deficient diets often find that they put on more weight they originally started with.

Proteins

Proteins are essential for growth and development. They provide the body with energy, and is needed for the manufacture of hormones, antibodies, enzymes, and tissues. Even though it sounds like just one substance, protein is actually a combination of many chemicals known as amino acids. There are 20 unique amino acids that make up protein, but they can combine in the body to make thousands of different proteins. Unlike fat cells for fat and muscle or liver for glucose, there is no place in the body to store protein. We need to consume enough protein to allow our muscles to be healthy and perform work. Of the 20 amino acids that are required for growth by the body, the human body can produce all but eight. These eight amino acids (essential) must be supplied to the body by food or supplements. The other 12 are referred to as nonessential amino acids. Whenever the body makes protein, while building muscle for instance-it needs a variety of amino acids for the protein-making process. These amino acids may come from dietary protein or from the body's own pool of amino acids. If a shortage of amino acids becomes chronic, which can occur if the diet is deficient in essential amino acids, the building of protein in the body stops, and the body suffers. It is very important for us to consume a full range of amino acids. And that's where balance and variety come into play.

Complete and Incomplete Proteins

Foods that contain all of the essential amino acids are called complete proteins. These foods include beef, chicken, fish, eggs, milk and just about anything else derived from animal sources; but soy and soy products also provide complete proteins. Incomplete proteins do not have all of the essential amino acids and generally include vegetables, fruits, grains, seeds and nuts.

So, if you're a vegetarian, to get all of the essential amino acids, mix and match foods from the following list:

barley • beans • Leafy greens • Corn meal • Lentils • sunflower seeds • broccoli • Oats • Peas • Nuts • rice • Peanuts • Cashews • Pasta • Whole grain breads

During normal exercise you only use protein for about 10% of your energy requirements. Most of the energy comes from carbohydrates and fats.

While exercising, you should eat more complex carbohydrates like cereals and grains in order to keep your body from breaking down protein for energy. Eating excessive protein is bad for your kidneys, liver, bones, cardiovascular system, and promotes vitamin and mineral deficiencies. It causes dehydration and is linked to osteoporosis, hypertension, and some forms of cancer. Despite popular belief, eating more protein will not help you make bigger muscles, unless you aren't eating enough protein. If you want to make your muscles bigger you need to give them appropriate stress and carbohydrates for fuel.

Protein Structure

Proteins are structurally composed of long chains of amino acids by peptide bonds. The order in which each the amino acids are linked together is called the primary structure. The primary structure dictates the final structure and function of the protein.

Protein Function

Proteins form the major structural components of muscle as well as that of the brain, nervous system, blood, skin, and hair. This important macronutrient serves as the transport mechanism for iron, vitamins, minerals, and oxygen within the body, and is the key to acid-base and fluid balance. Enzymes that speed up chemicals and antibodies that the body uses to fight infections are proteins. In situation of energy deprivation, the body can break down proteins for energy. With all of protein's essential functions, the human body is served well by consumption of the right kind and correct amount of high-quality proteins.

Protein Quality

A specific food's protein quality is determined by assessing its essential amino acid composition, digestibility and bioavailability. All proteins are made up of some combination of amino acid. There are nine essential amino acids, which, by definition, are amino acids that cannot be made by the body and must be consumed in the diet. The other eleven are called non-essential amino acids because they can be made by the body and can be made by the body and do not need to be obtained through the diet. Generally, animal products contain all of the essential amino acids (called complete proteins), whereas plant foods do not and are called incomplete proteins. However, there are notable exceptions such as buckwheat, chia seeds, flax seeds, hemp, quinoa, and soy, which are all plant-based complete proteins.

Another important thing to know about protein is its bioavailability. Protein bioavailability is the amount of protein the body can digest, absorb, and use. The more easily a protein – or any food for that matter – is digested, the more bioavailable it is to the body. Protein Digestibility-Corrected Amino Acid Score or PDCAAS is how the value of a protein is determined in the scientific world. That determination is based on both the amino acid requirements of humans and their ability to digest it. Animal proteins are complete proteins (have all essential amino acids), have higher PDCAAS values, and are therefore more bioavailable. That is why animal proteins are better sources of high-quality protein than plant proteins. However, an individual can boost protein quality and obtain all the essential amino acids by combining incomplete plant proteins to form a complementary protein. Excellent combinations include grains and legumes (rice and beans), grains and dairy (pasta and cheese), and legumes and seeds (falafel).

PROTEIN IS THE LEAST PREFERRED SOURCE OF ENERGY FOR THE BODY. THE USE OF PROTEIN FOR ENERGY RESULTS IN LOSS OF MUSCLE DENSITY, DECREASE IN STRENGTH, AND LOW IMMUNE SYSTEM.

Fats

Fats like everything else addressed in this book, "are not created equal". Many people treat fat like it is always a bad thing to be avoided at all cost. Actually, our bodies need some fat to function correctly. Fat insulates our bodies from the cold and provides some cushioning for our organs, it gives our bodies energy and helps to make up important hormones that we need to keep our bodies at the right temperature or keep our blood pressure at the right level.
Fat also helps in the creation of healthy skin and hair.

The fat that we consume is generally made up of the saturated fat and unsaturated fat:

• Saturated fat in most diets come from meat, milk, and milk products, but can also be found in poultry skin, coconut and palm oils, pastries, cookies.

• Unsaturated fat can be either monounsaturated or polyunsaturated. These fats come mostly from plant sources and are liquid at room temperature. Foods high in monounsaturated fat include avocados, olives, and peanuts. Canola, olive, almond, hazelnut, and peanut oils are also high in this type of fat. Foods high in polyunsaturated fat include fatty fish, nuts and vegetable oils such as safflower and sunflower.

Most dieticians and health professionals tell us to that in a healthy diet, we want to limit our saturated fat intake and we agree with them. Fat, whether from plant or animal sources, contains more than twice the number of calories of an equal amount of carbohydrate or protein. And, limited it will also help you lower your blood cholesterol level.

Fat Structure and Function

Lipids serve many important functions in the human body, including providing a readily available source of stored energy during times of caloric depravation, insulation, protection of vital organs and bones, a means for absorption of the fat-soluble vitamins, precursor to hormone, and cell membrane structure, among other necessary roles.

Sterols are a class of lipids that share a ring-like carbon structure. The most common sterile is cholesterol. Cholesterol is a fat-like, waxy substance produced in the liver and found in the cell membrane of all animal tissues, where it provides cell-structure and integrity. It is also found in that adrenal glands, testes and ovaries, and liver, where it forms the building blocks of the steroid hormones and bile acids.

Dietary fats consist mostly of triglycerides—a compound of three fatty acids attached to a glycerol (carbon and hydrogen structure) backbone. Triglycerides are the chemical form in which most fat exists in food as well as in the body. Fat is stored primarily as triglycerides and adipose tissue, providing a ready source of calories and energy in times of energy deprivation or fasting. Triglycerides also provide the body insulation (subcutaneous fat) and protection of vital organs (visceral fat) and bones (fat pad). Fat used to fuel exercise is mainly stored in the form of triglycerides in adipocytes (fat cells). A relatively small amount is also stored in muscle cells.

Fat as Fuel

Fats are the most concentrated source of energy, but only the second-best choice of energy for the body. The role of fat as an energy source is mainly determined by its availability to the muscle cell. To be metabolized, triglycerides must be broken down into FFAs and glycerol (via a process called lipolysis). As with carbohydrate usage, exercise intensity and duration determine which fat stores are used as fuel. During low-intensity exercise, circulating FFAs from adipocytes (i.e., plasma FFAs) are the primary source of fat energy. At higher intensities, metabolism of muscle triglycerides increases. Specifically, at exercise intensities indicated by great increase of breathing and heartbeats, the contribution of fat as a muscle fuel source is approximately equal between plasma FFAs and muscle triglycerides.

Vitamins, Minerals, and Water

Vitamins and minerals are the micronutrients that the body needs for energy production, immune function, blood clotting and other health benefits. Water has no nutrients and no calorie, but it's vital. Most people like to think of vitamins as drugs or some kind of medication. How many times have you heard the phrase: I'm going take more vitamin C because I feel a little under the weather? Problem is, it's too late at that point. See, unlike drugs, vitamins do not have you any "immediate effects" and swallowing a few pills of vitamins would make any difference. So, you need to take your vitamins just like foods (regularly and at the right dosage). There is a long list of vitamins to know about. Here are some of them and their functions:

- **Vitamin A (retinol):** Retinol has multiple has multiple functions. It is essential for vision, skin and mucous membranes, cells growth, reproduction, and normal immunity.

- **Vitamin b1 (Thiamin):** Thiamin (thiamine is a water-soluble vitamin that enters and leaves the body daily. Vitamin B1 helps maintain normal energy metabolism. Thiamin is required for the oxidative decarboxylation of alpha-keto acids and for transketlase activity in the pentose phosphate pathway, Thiamin works to burn carbs.

- **Vitamin b2 (riboflavin):** Riboflavin helps the mitochondria (furnaces) of your muscle cells produce energy. Meats, poultry, fish, and dairy products are all good food sources.

- **Vitamin b3 (Niacin, Niacinamide):** Niacin is another water-soluble vitamin partly supplied by the tryptophan in your diet, which the body converts to niacin. It functions as part of two enzymes, nicotinamide adenine dinucleothide, and with an additional phosphate.

- **Vitamin b6 (Pyridoxine):** Pyridoxine coenzymes functions at all levels of protein and amino acid metabolism, and in making of hemoglobin and all new proteins. It is also essential for the enzyme glycogen phosphorylase that breaks down muscle glycogen for fuel. So the right amount of vitamins B6 is very important to athletes.

- **Pantothenic Acid (Vitamin b5):** B-complex of water-soluble vitamins that have multiple roles in energy metabolism. It forms part of the important coenzyme A, and part of one of the carries proteins for the enzyme fatty acid synthetase.

- **Folate (Folic Acid, Folacin):** A B-complex that forms part of natal transports coenzymes that control amino acid metabolism. An insufficiency of Folate inhibits growth of new cells.

- **Vitamin b12 (Cyanocobalamin):** Cobalamin forms part of coenzymes essential for al cells, particularly rapid –turnover cells, including red blood cells, the lining of the gastrointestinal tract, and bone marrow cells. Deficiency of vitamins B12 causes pernicious anemia, which wipes out your nerves and sends you raving mad before killing you. This B-complex vitamin is available only in animal foods. Vegetarians are the most commonly deficient.

- **Biotin:** Biotin is the least of the B-complex vitamins. By forming part of two enzymes, pyruvate carboxylase, and acetyl-coenzyme. A carboxylase, biotin is essential for gluconeogenesis (formation of new glucose) and fatty acid synthesis.

- **Vitamin C (Ascorbate):** Like the B-complex, vitamin C is water soluble (except for the ascorbyl palmitate form), and quickly in and out of the body.

- **Vitamin D (Cholecalciferol):** Vitamin D is essential for bone growth and mineral balance in our body.

- **Vitamin E (D-alpha-tocopherol):** The main function of vitamin E is as an antioxidant.

- **Vitamin K (Phylloquinone):** The last of the fat-soluble vitamins, phylloquinone is essential for formation of prothrombin one of the compounds that enables blood to clot.

VITAMINS A, D, E, AND K ARE FAT-SOLUBLE, ALL OTHER VITAMINS ARE WATER-SOLUBLE.

Minerals are "the framework" of our health. Here are a few of them and their functions.

• **Calcium:** About 99% of your 3lbs. (1.4kg) or so of calcium is built into your bones. The remaining 1% circulates around, involved in myriad functions from conduction of nerve impulses to contraction of muscles.

• **Phosphorus:** Adenosine Tri-phosphate (ATP), your basic energy compound consists of one molecule of adenosine bonded to three molecules of phosphate. One of these phosphate molecules used up as ATP is converted to energy. The ATP is then regenerated by a phosphate molecule taken from Creatine Phosphate stored in the muscle.

• **Potassium:** Three main electrolytes responsible for the flow of electromagnetic energy: potassium, sodium and chloride. Potassium is the most important.

• **Sulfur:** Is essential for everything from use of B-vitamins, to blood coagulation, immune function, antioxidant defenses, and the maintenance of the lining of your heart.

• **Magnesium:** 60% of the body's magnesium resides in your bones. 40% is essential for all body manufacturing processes, burning of glycogen for fuel, transmission of the genetic code to form new proteins, and the activity of over 300 enzymes.

• **Iron:** Hemoglobin is the red pigment in blood that extracts oxygen from the air in your lungs, and delivers it to your muscles, organs and brain. Production of hemoglobin largely depends on your body's use of iron.

• **Zinc:** Is essential for all cell growth and forms part of numerous enzymes in every animal and every plant on Earth. The pool of available zinc in the human body is small and rapidly used so it has to be replaced daily.

• **Iodine:** Forms part of your thyroid hormones, thyroxine and triodothyronine. Because your thyroid is a major controller of energy processes, you better get enough of it.

• **Chromium:** Is essential for insulin metabolism. Because of its potentiation of insulin, chromium was established as an essential element for carbohydrate, fat and protein metabolism, glucose control and muscle growth.

The Truth About Water

Incredible as it may seem, water is quite possible the single most important catalyst in losing weight and keeping it off. Although most of us take it for granted, water may be the only true "magic potion" for permanent weight-management and a healthy lifestyle too!

How Water Can Affect Fat-Loss

Water suppresses the appetite naturally and helps the body metabolize stored fat. Studies show that a decrease in water intake will cause fat deposits to increase, while an increase in water can actually reduce deposits.

H2O Awesome!

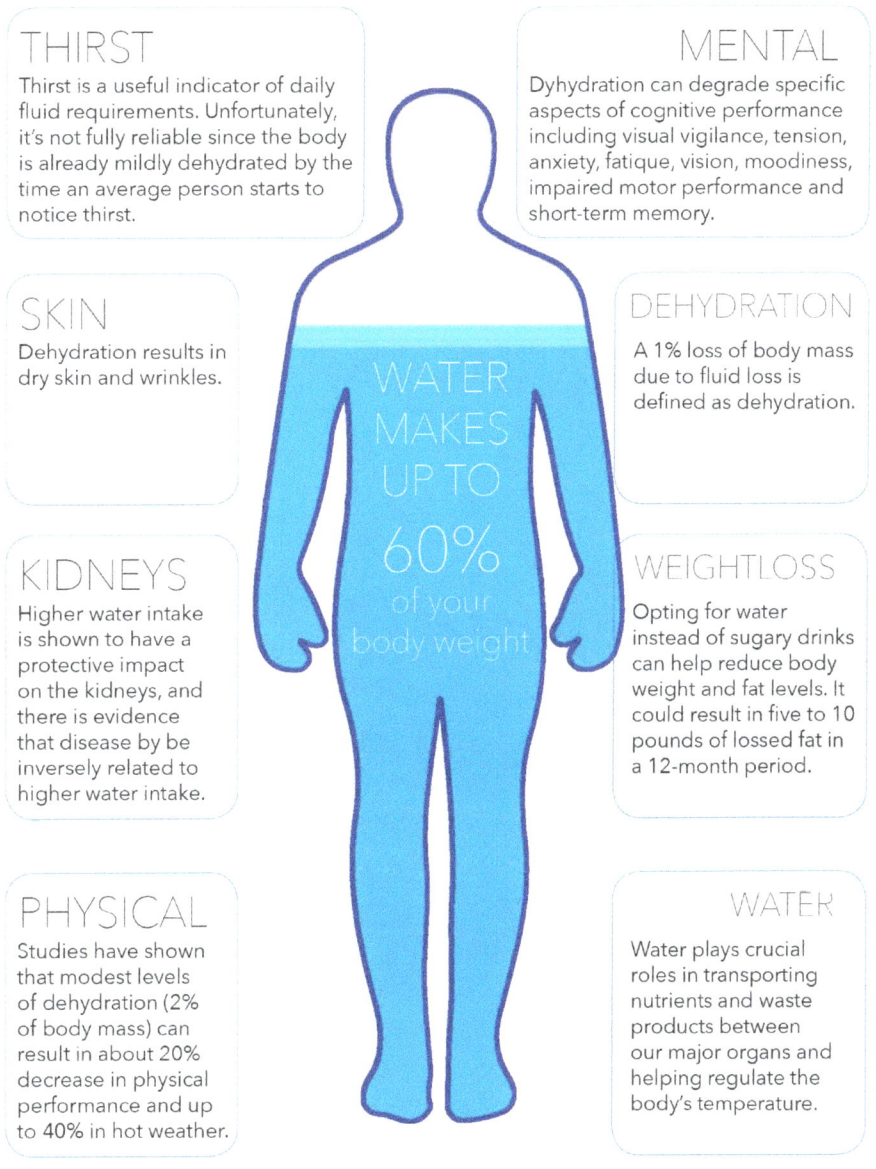

THIRST
Thirst is a useful indicator of daily fluid requirements. Unfortunately, it's not fully reliable since the body is already mildly dehydrated by the time an average person starts to notice thirst.

MENTAL
Dyhydration can degrade specific aspects of cognitive performance including visual vigilance, tension, anxiety, fatique, vision, moodiness, impaired motor performance and short-term memory.

SKIN
Dehydration results in dry skin and wrinkles.

DEHYDRATION
A 1% loss of body mass due to fluid loss is defined as dehydration.

WATER MAKES UP TO 60% of your body weight

KIDNEYS
Higher water intake is shown to have a protective impact on the kidneys, and there is evidence that disease by be inversely related to higher water intake.

WEIGHTLOSS
Opting for water instead of sugary drinks can help reduce body weight and fat levels. It could result in five to 10 pounds of lossed fat in a 12-month period.

PHYSICAL
Studies have shown that modest levels of dehydration (2% of body mass) can result in about 20% decrease in physical performance and up to 40% in hot weather.

WATER
Water plays crucial roles in transporting nutrients and waste products between our major organs and helping regulate the body's temperature.

Why? The kidneys can't function properly without enough water. When the kidneys don't function to capacity, some of the workload is taken on by the liver. The liver's primary function is to metabolize stored fat into usable energy. If the liver has to do some of the kidney's work, it can't function at its optimal capacity. As a result, it metabolizes less fat. More fat remains stored and weight-loss/fat-loss stops.

The best way to overcome water retention is to give the body more water. The body will then release the stored water.

Diuretics offer only temporary relief of water retention. Your body will perceive this as a threat to survival and hold on to every drop. If you have a constant problem with water retention, excess salt may be your problem. The more salt you eat the more water your body will hold. It holds onto water to dilute the salt because the body can only tolerate so much sodium.

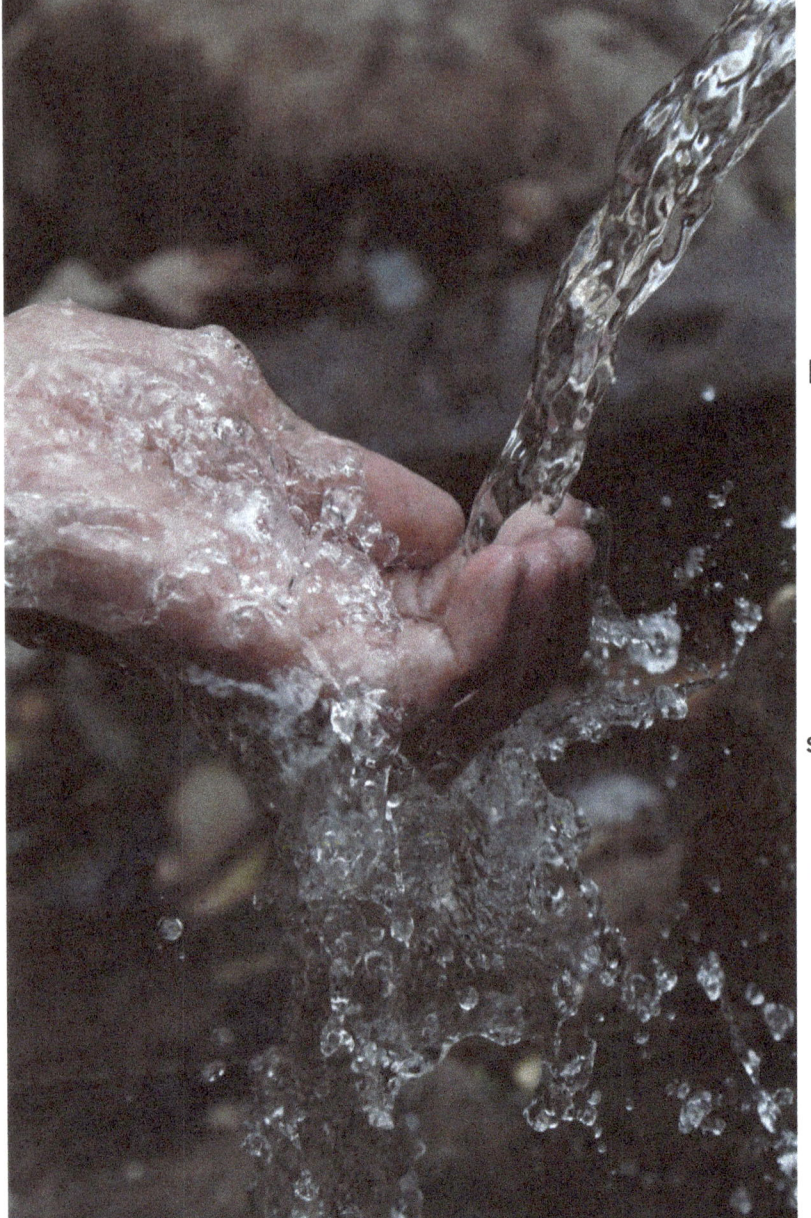

To get rid of sodium, drink more water. Water will remove sodium as it passes through the kidneys.

Water contributes greatly to the natural ability of the muscle to contract by preventing dehydration, for muscles are primarily made up of water.

How much water is enough?

On the average and sedentary person should drink at least 8 glasses of glasses of water a day. The overweight person needs one additional glass for every 25 pounds of excess weight.

5 Weight Management Facts

• The commercial weight-loss market generates over $36 billion each year. How? Repeat business.

• Conventional weight-loss programs experience a 98% failure rate. Why? Because people lose lean muscle, not fat. Once they resume normal eating habits...the weight returns, plus more.

• You can't starve fat off your body. Why? Fat doesn't need to be fed. Since prehistoric times, the

• The "cure all" diet is a hoax. Why? Everyone is genetically different. Everyone processes food differently. You are unique.

• Proper nutrition, productive exercise, and positive motivation is the only valid technique to achieve long-term weight-management. Why? Without exercise supported by nutrition and motivation, you will more likely lose muscle, not fat.

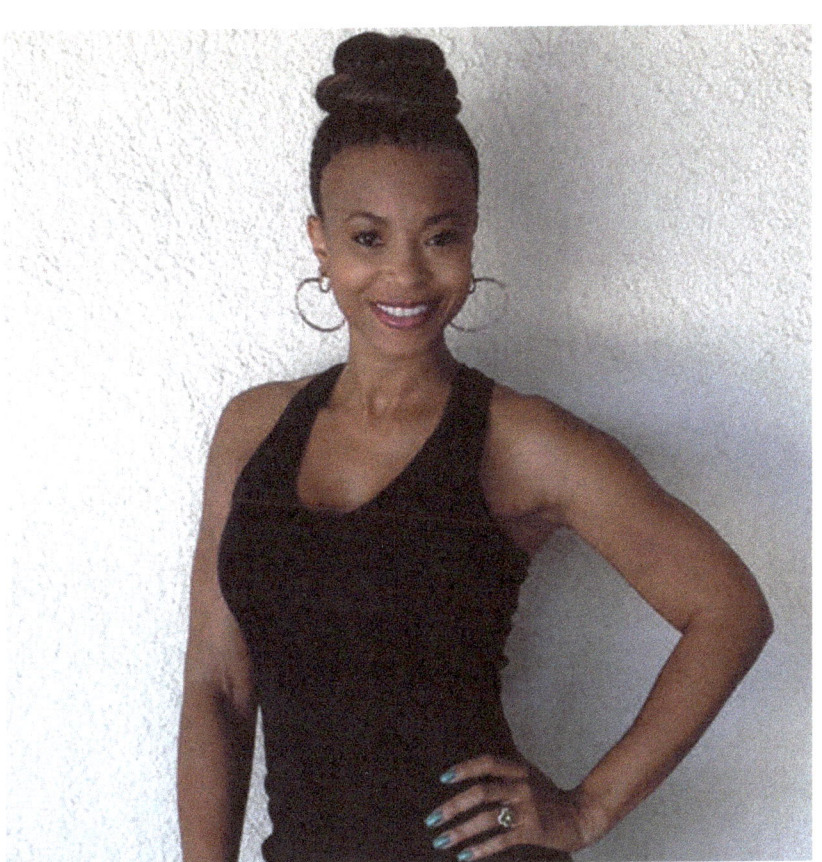

The Power of Protein

Focus on eating protein and vegetables, which as you can see from the lists of acceptable foods in the Food List offer you a remarkable array of choices. In addition to the palm-size portions of protein you'll eat at each meal-yes, big-handed guys get more than small-handed gals-you'll be eating plenty of leafy green vegetables and two snacks of seeds or nuts. And in place of these palm-size portions of meat, poultry, fish, and meat substitutes, you can also have the following servings of protein:

- 1 cup of fresh cheese, such as cottage or ricotta
- 1ounce of aged cheeses, such as Cheddar or Swiss
- 1 cup of plain unsweetened yogurt
- 1 cup of plain or flavored unsweetened soymilk
- 1 cup of plain or flavored unsweetened almond milk
- 2 or 3 eggs (preferably omega-3 and free-range), up to 4 per day
- ½ cup black soybeans (not to be confused with black beans) or edamame (green soybeans)
- 1 package of shirataki tofu noodles.

The Failure Cycle

Conventional diets don't work because they are faulty in design. They are based on weight-loss instead of fat loss. You restrict yourself to a very low-calorie diet or liquid diet and think you are reaching your goal because you are losing weight. But, because that diet is not designed to lose fat, you are mainly losing muscle weight. Consequently, upon resuming normal eating habits, you gain the weight back. So, as they cycle goes you start the same method all over again – only to fail once more. It's called yo-yo dieting.

The Key to permanent weight-management is understanding

the difference between weight-loss and fat-loss.

You are not alone – according to the National Institute of Health, almost 98% of dieters gain their original weight back, plus more. People on liquid diets realize, only after their programs are over, they are no more prepared to face real food again then they were before their programs started.

Don't be Too Concerned with Your scale

In almost all conventional diet programs, the weight you lose is mainly muscle. Therefore, you only become a smaller version of yourself – a skinnier FAT person. Your body fat percentage hardly changes. But, your bathroom scale would have you believe a conventional diet really works.
In fact, if you are on a good weight-management program that includes strength training to build lean muscle mass, you weight will initially INCREASE. That's right. You are adding muscle, and muscle weighs more than fat. Many may quit a program that's working, because they don't understand the process is actually doing what it is designed to do.

Humans are built for survival! So, why do we retain body-fat? The answer goes back thousands and thousands of years. Early humans ate anything and everything they could. They instinctively did so because it might be days or even weeks before they found another good source of food if any. To survive, the body stored as much fat as possible to be burned as fat later. That is even more so for women because of their reproductive and child-bearing abilities. We have not evolved from this state. We still are efficient fat-storing machines. The built-in survival mechanism is strong. Your body continually makes instinctive adjustments to stay alive. Dieting is no exception. In your mind, you know you are simply dieting, – however, your body believes you are starving to death – and instinctively seeks high-calorie food in order to store and hoard fat.

Exercise Lowers Your Fat Thermostat

In order to lose fat permanently, your fat thermostat must be lowered. You'll need to convince your body to burn fat instead of muscle. By doing so, your weight-loss will be fat-loss. Lowering your fat thermostat also will increase your metabolic rate (which is good) as you begin to lose improper food cravings.

The Truth

It's a medical fact. There's no such thing as a universal formula that works for everybody. You must learn how your body works and how you will burn fat instead of muscle. It is the only way you'll lose fat and fain permanent control of your weight.

However, there are three basic steps to permanent fat-loss. They include:

1. Optimal Calorie Intake: It's important to identify the optimal calorie intake you need by quantifying and qualifying variables in your body such as height, weight, gender, body-fat level, muscle tissue, activity level and genetic traits.

2. Exercise: Oxygen is imperative in order to optimally burn fat. Therefore, cardiovascular activity is essential. In addition, exercise sends a message to your body that muscle is more valuable than fat. Exercise can be a brisk walk or as intense as aerobics and/or weight training. Exercise depends on your personal goals and current physical condition. Through exercise, you teach your body to keep muscle. Therefore, it must burn fat for energy.

3. Motivation: In the final analysis, weight-management is up to you. You can continue on the failure cycle or, make a long-term commitment to better health. If you chose the latter, there is only one way -– proper nutrition and exercise.

Here are some easy eating tips and ideas:

• Try to drink eight 8 oz. glasses of water per day.

• Many liquids contain calories. Good examples are Gatorade, fruit juices and flavored water.

• Be sure to read labels. Sometimes understanding labels can be tricky.

• Remember, sugar comes in many different forms, corn syrup, honey, sucrose, dextrose, maltose, and galactose. Be aware of words ending in "ose."

• Fructose is the most preferred source of sugar (not fructose syrup or high fructose corn syrup).

• Always use fresh whole fruits and vegetables whenever possible. Use frozen fruit and vegetables as a second choice. When fruits and vegetables are canned, up to 90% of certain vitamins and minerals might be lost in the process.

• Sweeten your oatmeal with naturally sweeten jams (no artificial sugars/high-fructose syrup).

• Spice up your air-popped popcorn with Tabasco, salsa, or other non-fattening spices.

• Try the following foods on top of your potato: low fat or nonfat cottage cheese, nonfat cheese, non-fat salad dressing, non-fat sour cream or fresh salsa. Boil your rice water with a bouillon cube. Try your favorite non-fat dressing on fresh steamed vegetables.

• Have a whole wheat (or pita) burrito instead of chicken and rice. Use the following ingredients: fresh tortilla, lean ground meats, vegetables, non-fat beans, non-fat cheese and fresh salsa.

• Instead of syrup and butter on pancakes, try natural apple butter, fruit puree, or non-fat yogurt.

• Use non-fat cheese or non-fat Ricotta as a substitute for regular cheese.

• Use salsa or Balsamic vinegar on salads instead of regular dressing.

YOUR BODY'S DEFENSE MECHANISM AGAINST DIETING OR STARVATION

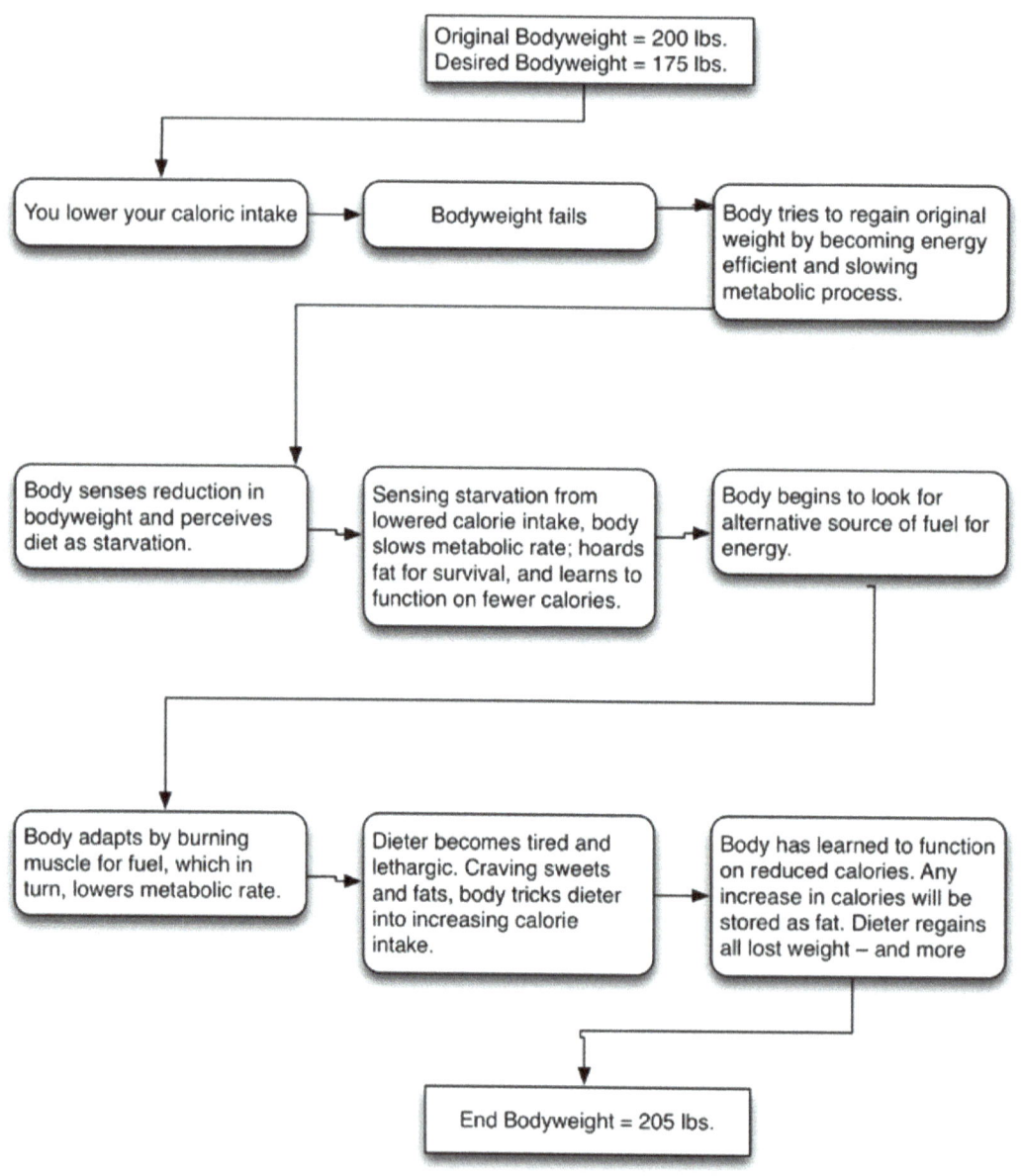

This is the unavoidable result of restricted calorie diets, "quick-fix" diets or liquid diet programs. If you feel you need to take your weight-management to the next logical level, or just don't want to manage the entire process alone, consult with a nutritionist or a registered dietitian in your local area.

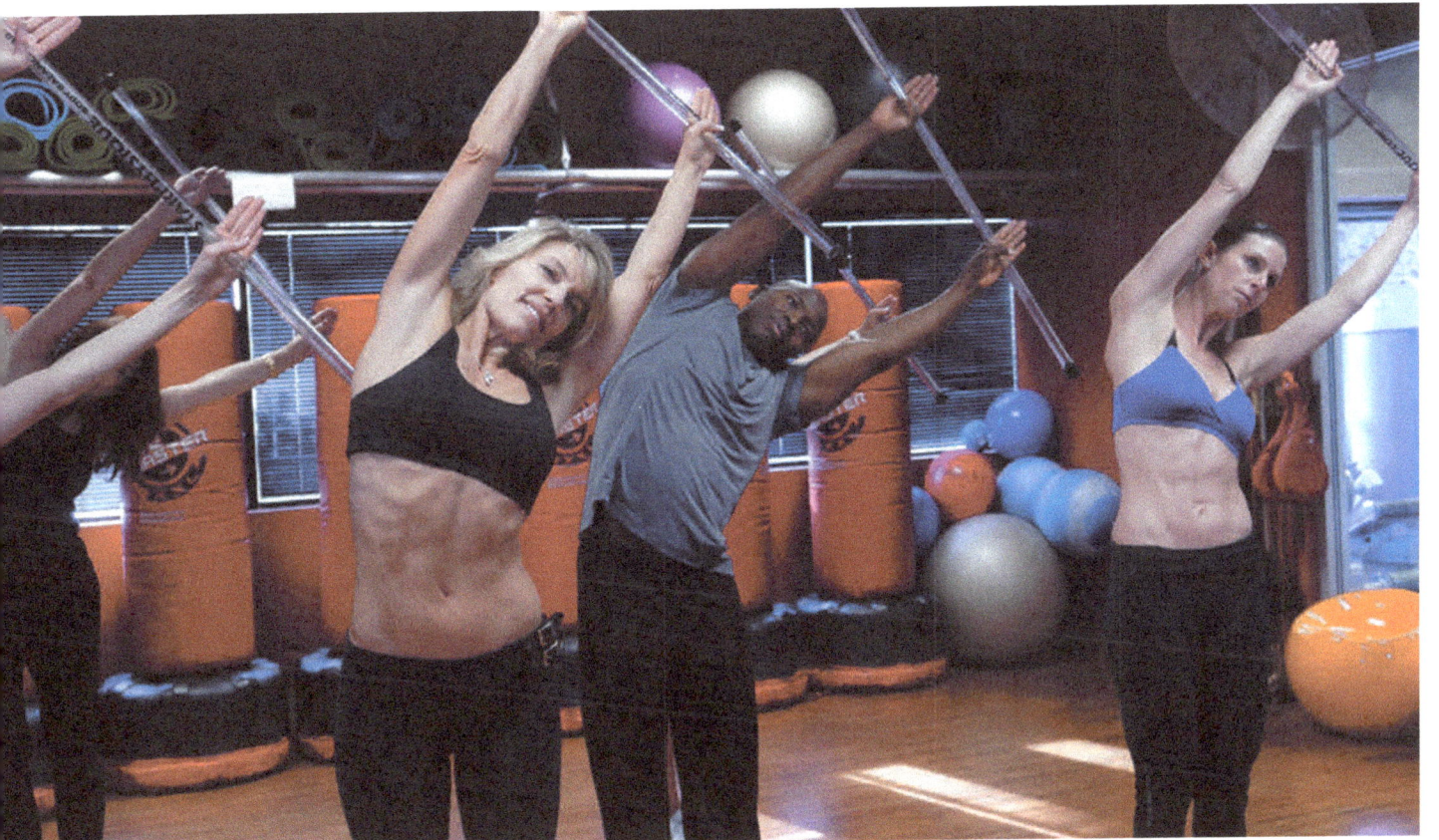

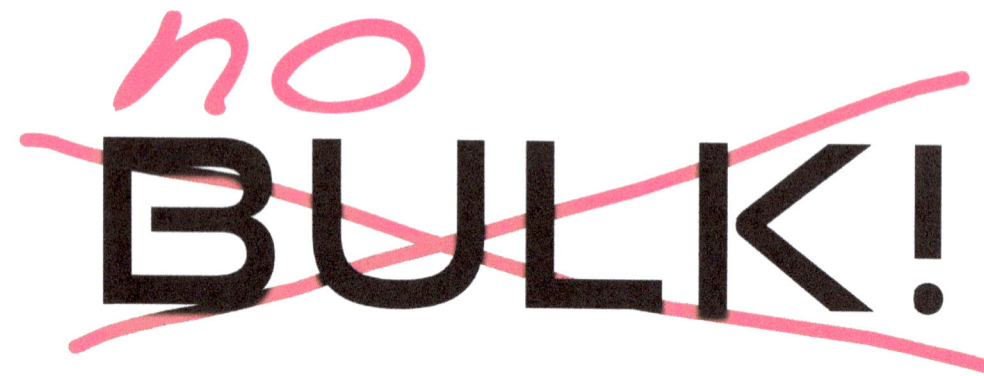

No Warranty

G Power Productions, LLC. does not guarantee the accuracy, completeness, timeliness or correct sequencing of any of the Information in this manual, including, but not limited to Information originated by Garba "Mister G" Onadja, licensed by G Power Productions, LLC. or gathered by G Power Productions, LLC from publicly available sources.

G POWER PRODUCTIONS, LLC. MAKES NO REPRESENTATIONS OR WARRANTIES, WHETHER EXPRESS OR IMPLIED, ABOUT THE SUITABILITY OF THE INFORMATION, SOFTWARE, PRODUCTS OR SERVICES CONTAINED IN THIS MANUAL. ALL SUCH INFORMATION, SOFTWARE, PRODUCTS AND SERVICES ARE PROVIDED "AS IS" WITHOUT WARRANTY OF ANY KIND.

No Liability

G POWER PRODUCTIONS, LLC. SHALL HAVE NO LIABILITY, CONTINGENT OR OTHERWISE, FOR THE ACCURACY, COMPLETENESS, TIMELINESS OR CORRECT SEQUENCING OF THE INFORMATION OR FOR ANY DECISION MADE OR ACTION TAKEN BY YOU IN RELIANCE UPON THE INFORMATION IN THIS MANUAL.

Making You **StrongSleekFit!**

*"I was so amazed by the power of
gTonnicks's The Sleekest Workout that I recruited all my friends
to try some of the moves. In less than three weeks,
The Sleekest Workout™ improved my body and my athleticism!"*

– Amir Ahmadian, 7-foot tall aspiring pro-basketball player

ABOUT THE AUTHOR

Garba "Mister G" Onadja is considered the Calabasas Top Personal Trainer & Fitness Motivator. Born in Niger, West Africa, Mister G grew up as one of the country's most popular high school and collegiate athletes. He was also selected to represent West Africa on its National Taekwondo Exhibition Team for the Seoul 1988 Olympics. His success and popularity landed him a job as a body conditioning and self-defense instructor for U.S. Marine Security Guard in Niger, West Africa before he left to live and study in France. While living in France, he found himself training in St. Lauren DuVar, a small town near the French Riviera popular for both Ballet and La Savate, the French form of kickboxing. During this time, Mister G started to notice how La Savate and Ballet both utilized similar movements to strengthen and perfect their execution and reasoned that: "if changed ever so slightly and performed precisely, these movements could be used to tone and strengthen nearly any part of the body". In that moment, his vision for gTonnicks (www.TheSleeKestWorkout.com or www.gTonnickStyle.com), an elegant approach to fitness, toning and strength development, was born. In 2004 he was inducted into the USA Martial Arts Hall of Fame. And, although he has been honored many times professionally, he considers the L.A.Daily News' readers naming him: "the most motivational instructor" in the Valley, among his most prized recognitions.

NO weights and NO machines! Just your body and the gBalance Bar. The movements are simple, but don't be fooled, they are the kind of movements that will make your muscles scream and leave you at awe and raving about it. And then, you will truly understand why "The Body Is The Best Machine!"

-Garba "Mister G." Onadja

info@gpowercreations.com • www.TheSleekestWorkout.com • www.gTonnickStyle.com